COOK
This
NOW

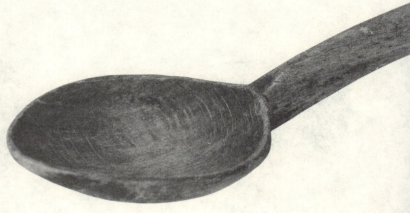

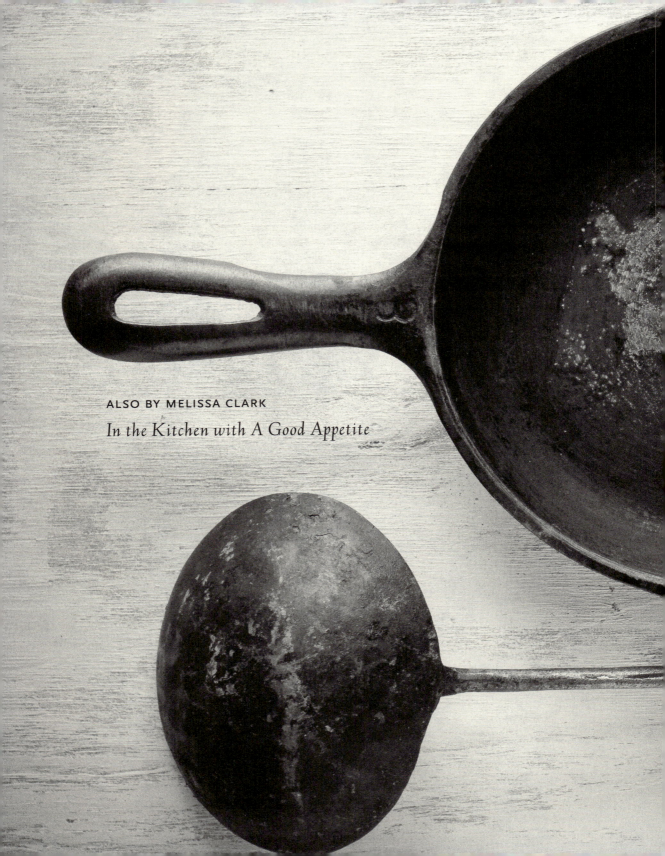

ALSO BY MELISSA CLARK

In the Kitchen with A Good Appetite

COOK
This
NOW

120 EASY AND DELECTABLE DISHES
YOU CAN'T WAIT TO MAKE

Melissa Clark

HYPERION
NEW YORK

Library of Congress Cataloging-in-Publication Data

Clark, Melissa.
    Cook this now : 120 easy and delectable dishes you can't wait to make / Melissa Clark. — 1st ed.
        p. cm.
    Includes index.
    ISBN 978-1-4013-2398-1 (hardback)
  1. Cooking, American. 2. Cookbooks. I. Title. II. Title: 120 easy and delectable dishes you can't wait to make.
    TX715.C57787 2011
    641.5973—dc22

                                                                2011010420

Hyperion books are available for special promotions and premiums. For details contact the HarperCollins Special Markets Department in the New York office at 212-207-7528, fax 212-207-7222, or email spsales@harpercollins.com.

Book design by Shubhani Sarkar

Color photography by Andrew Scrivani

FIRST EDITION

10   9   8   7   6   5   4   3   2   1

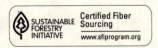

THIS LABEL APPLIES TO TEXT STOCK

We try to produce the most beautiful books possible, and we are also extremely concerned about the impact of our manufacturing process on the forests of the world and the environment as a whole. Accordingly, we've made sure that all of the paper we use has been certified as coming from forests that are managed, to ensure the protection of the people and wildlife dependent upon them.

For Daniel and Dahlia,
who sustain me,
every season of the year

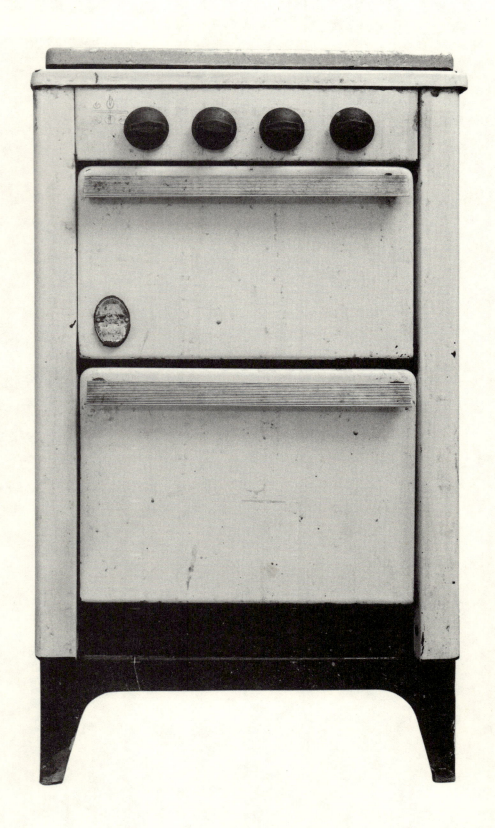

Contents

MARCH

Spring

APRIL

MAY

JUNE

Summer

JULY

AUGUST

SEPTEMBER

Autumn

DECEMBER

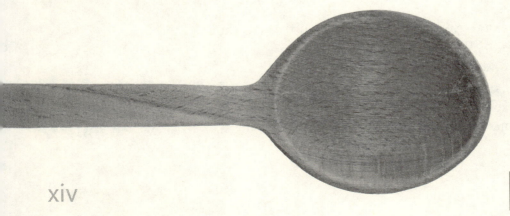

Bonus Recipes

FROM MELISSA CLARK'S COOKBOOK *In the Kitchen with A Good Appetite*

Photographs follow pages 140 and 332.

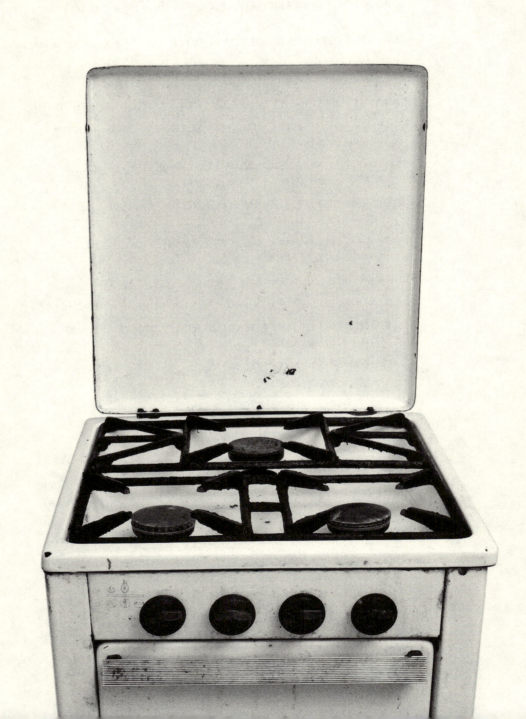

Acknowledgments

As usual, creating a book is a collaborative experience, and there are many people to thank. First off, a big thank-you goes out to my fantastic Hyperion team, including my editor Leslie Wells, Elisabeth Dyssegaard, publisher Ellen Archer, and their intrepid design gurus Laura Klynstra and Shubhani Sarkar.

Thanks to my pal Andrew Scrivani for the stunning photos made even more lavish by the incredible food and prop styling of Soo Jeong Kang, with essential help from Olga Massov.

Once again, I am exceedingly grateful to my literary agent Janis Donnaud, who is always ahead of whatever game she's in. I couldn't even begin to do what I do without her. A whipped cream mountain of thanks to my loyal recipe testers and trusted friends Sarah Huck and Jaimee Young, who help make my days happier and brighter and easier on so many important levels. Thanks to my tireless book publicist, Carrie Bachman, who is stellar at getting the word out.

A giant thankful hug to my longtime friend and past collaborator Robin Aronson for pitching in at the last minute to get this book finished—reading text, line editing, testing recipes, giving general feedback and support. I can't imagine actually having finished this manuscript without Robin's help.

And thanks to Kate Krader, who came up with the brilliant alternate title "A Year of Excellent Eating." And to my friends who were always willing to listen to my book-related ramblings and anxieties whenever I couldn't bear to keep them to myself, including Alice Feiring, Frank Bruni, Susan Gross, Karen Rush, Dave Wondrich (who also helped with lots of punch), Kate Heddings, Josh Mack, Bryony Romer, Ana Deboo, Sara Kate Gillingham-Ryan, Shawn Kelley, John Magazino, and Zoe Singer.

To all the farmers at New York City farmers' markets who inspire me with the bounty of their stalls in every season, even in the frozen winter, I thank you. And to all the WiFi-equipped cafes in Prospect Heights, thanks for the countless cups of tea that fueled my writing.

Thank you, as always, to my parents and sister for all their support, honest opinions, and for taking home lots of leftovers.

And finally, there's no adequate way to thank my husband Daniel and daughter Dahlia, for what turned out to be sacrifices to our family life during the writing of this book, which was on a tight schedule. If I were somehow able to stitch three more months into the fabric of last year, I would. Instead a heartfelt thank-you will have to do, offered with heaps of love.

COOK
This
NOW

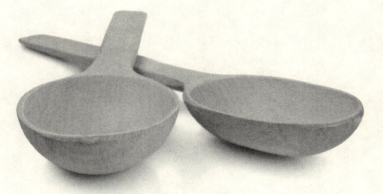

Winter

In winter, Brooklyn's Grand Army Plaza farmers' market is strictly for the hard core. The wind shoots mercilessly across the park and some mornings are so frigid that the milk we just bought stipples with ice as it bumps along in the bottom of the stroller. A damp, bitter cold invades your bones and burns the skin on your fingertips the second you take your gloves off to sort through a half-frozen mound of spinach in order to gather a small pile of unwilted leaves.

But I go almost every week, wrapping myself in sweaters and scarves and knee-length down coat. My daughter, Dahlia, gets the cocoon treatment, first zipped into a snowsuit, then into bunting, before being sealed in beneath a windproof plastic liner. Even so, when she bites off her mittens, her hands glow red in minutes. Oddly, Daniel, my husband, wears a leather jacket and no gloves, but he has a whole other kind of metabolism going on.

Trudging through the cold to wander the relatively barren farm stands definitely feels a little nuts when instead, nestled on the couch with my steaming tea and hot, buttered toast, I can order pretty much whatever I want with a quick click to my local online grocer.

But I go nonetheless—even on the dampest, windiest, grayest, most foul mornings—because, well, I like it.

I like the farmers, sleepily zombie-like in their coveralls and parkas, hopping side to side to stay warm. The quietness of the cold gives us an opportunity for conversation, and now is the time to seek out their advice on everything from celery root trimming to mulching, chatter that the busier seasons don't allow.

I like the other shoppers, as freezing and obsessed as I am, with their dogs and kids and spouses in tow, breathing steam into the air. It's a quirky winter community of diehards, a loosely knit group connected by a quest for the tastiest collard greens, the perkiest parsnips.

But maybe most important, I like the way my weekly trips ground me in the seasons. It's one thing to know intellectually that in January, turnips are in season (or in storage) and zucchini is not. But it is another thing entirely to experience the limits firsthand, and to settle into them, accepting them as winter's inevitabilities, like 4:00 P.M. sunsets and salt stains on leather boots.

In a way it's a little like moving from the big city of summer produce—with a population so vast it's impossible to know everyone's name (what exactly are those little yellow plums called?)—to the small town of winter, where the occupants are few and you can get to know them and all their charms and quirks intimately. I don't know that I would have fallen as hard for rutabagas if I hadn't bought them, week in and week out, from December to April. But now I'm completely smitten with their velvety, pumpkin-like flesh.

Actually, now that I know it so well, I can honestly say I'm a little in love with winter's bounty—even if I can name the offerings on all my fingers and toes. My kitchen diary lists the typical winter haul: apples, some crisp and juicy for immediate snacking, some mealy and soft to make into applesauce. Kale, often yellowed around the crinkled edges but still succulent and green-tasting, just begs for a braise spiked with anchovies and pecorino (page 12). The collards, with sweet, green-black leaves as thick as leather, are best boiled, then dressed with lemon and plenty of good olive oil (page 83). Pale heads of cabbage as big and heavy as bowling balls may be borscht bound (page 348) or roasted (page 88). I keep the kohlrabi for snacking on raw, sweet as carrots but running with juice. Golden and purple turnips with delicate pale flesh and waxy rutabaga are perfect for roasting with the market's treacly maple syrup (page 361). Hairy celery roots get whittled down for crunchy salads, punctuated by roasted hazelnuts and bitter arugula (page 40). Dark orange sweet potatoes are to bake in their jackets until the juices seep out and turn sticky. There are eggs with marigold yolks, and creamy-topped milk from contented but probably very cold cows.

Even when the ground is iced over with nothing new peeping out for months, the possibility of discovery is always there, lurking next to the onions. Sometimes I snag a treat. Once it was frozen summer heirloom tomatoes from farmer Ray Bradley. I bought four large ones to melt into pasta sauce with rosemary and his bacon, a wintry version of a sauce that I usually save for September (page 262). Another week, he had frozen raspberries that Dahlia and I ate with local yogurt and more of that thick maple syrup.

You never know what the meat guys are going to show up with, and I love the challenge of experimenting with cuts not usually seen in the supermarket. I've bought everything from oxtails to turkey necks to smoked ham hocks—then figured out what to do with them after I got home.

Once, I picked up a pair of pig's feet, expecting four pink, neatly sliced halves that had been defurred, blanched, bleached, and well cleaned, the toenails manicured off. That's the rather sterilized product you get at the supermarket.

These feet were about as close to the source as I'd ever come—whole and intact, muddy toenails and all, with a thick coat of dark brown and gray mottled bristles covering the flesh.

I spent hours on the Internet and Twitter trying to figure out how to handle them.

"Blanch them in boiling water, then scrape the hair off with the back of a knife."

"Singe the bristles off with a blowtorch but open the window first—burning pig fur stinks."

"Shave the trotters with a razor—or several."

I dallied so long trying to decide what to do that the feet festered in the fridge and I had to throw them out. I can't say I wasn't relieved.

Compared to this, the oxtails were a breeze. I seared them until bronzed, then braised them with port and red wine until the meat was short ribs–succulent and falling off the bone, enveloped in a brawny, glossy gravy (page 25). Then we ate them with roasted turnips and potatoes (page 29).

Of course my trips to the market in winter are shorter and more to the point than during the rest of the year. There is no socializing with other parents-with-toddlers on a grassy patch at the mouth of the park. Not much chatting about what's about to come into season, because for months, the answer is the same: nothing much. No comparing recipes for celery root because after weeks (even years) of prior discussions, all the regulars know each other's tricks by now.

Instead we go, we shop, we shiver, we come home, we unpack our minimal yet cherished spoils, and make yet another pot of tea to thaw the icicles out of our bloodstreams.

Sometimes, after a particularly frigid Saturday morning trip to the farmers' market, we don't leave the house for the rest of the day. We've had our exercise, communed with the outside world, schlepped home our food for the week. We feel we've earned the right to stay in, warm and cozy, reading Frog and Toad books to Dahlia on the couch while watching the little bit of sky that we can see from our window change from washed-out blue to white to black night.

And all the while, we cook. Whether it's baked apple crisp covered in cardamom-scented crumbs in the oven (page 31) or garlicky, herb-scented, long-simmered cannellini beans on the stove (page 8), in winter the kitchen is always alive, always warm, always inviting me in for just one more cup of hot tea.

JANUARY

WHITE BEAN STEW WITH ROSEMARY, GARLIC, AND FARRO

There are few things as reassuring as having a pot of something good to eat bubbling away on the stove when you're home on a chilly afternoon. What's actually in the pot almost doesn't matter. The simmering sound and steamy scent will cheer you on bleak days. And having a pot going will make you feel productive, despite the fact that you're not actually doing anything. This is especially true of beans, which will transform from hard and pebble-like to soft and supple all by themselves, without any poking and prodding and stirring from you. Just season the pot, turn on the heat, and get out of the way. Go answer e-mails on the couch, and when you come back later, dinner will be done.

I make countless variations on a basic bean stew all winter long and never get tired of it. It's comfort food, but it offers a complex comfort, more interesting than, say, mashed potatoes, and more sophisticated and unexpected than macaroni and cheese or even roast chicken.

This version, steeped with piney rosemary, good, grassy olive oil, and plenty of garlic, reminds me of Tuscany, where everything is similarly perfumed. Once, I spent a week there writing an article about a cooking school held in a Renaissance villa. One day I stood in the big, rustic kitchen, openmouthed in awe as the cook upended an entire bottle of last year's olive oil into the bean pot. She needed to use it up to make way for the new oil, which was being pressed. Those might have been the best beans I've ever had, and though I am liberal with my olive oil anointing, it is a mere drizzle compared with hers.

I usually serve my bean pot with some kind of sautéed green because I like the contrast both in color (pale beige/bright green) and flavor (earthy, rich, and mild compared to silky, garlicky, and grassy). Tuscan kale is my favorite here because of my happy Italian associations, but collards, mustard greens, regular kale, and spinach are also splendid and generally available all winter long. And serving the beans with a grain, such as the nutty, chewy farro, adds a textural contrast and makes the bean pot a perfect protein unto itself.

I still haven't been able to get my toddler, Dahlia, to eat more than a bean or two at a time. But she adores the bean broth, which she drinks with a straw. I don't know what they would say about that in Tuscany.

Serves 6

1 pound dried cannellini beans

1/4 cup extra-virgin olive oil, more for drizzling

5 garlic cloves, peeled

1 celery stalk, cut in half crosswise (reserve the celery leaves for garnishing)

1 large onion, halved lengthwise from root to stem so it holds together

1 whole clove (stick it in the onion half)

2 rosemary sprigs

2 thyme sprigs

1 bay leaf

Piece of Parmesan rind, if you like

2 1/2 teaspoons kosher or coarse sea salt, more to taste

1 cup farro, rinsed (see What Else?)

Flaky salt, such as Maldon or fleur de sel

1/4 teaspoon Turkish or Syrian red pepper such as Urfa, Maras, or Aleppo

Chopped celery or parsley leaves, for garnish (optional)

Lemon juice and/or grated Parmesan cheese, for serving (optional)

1. If you have the time and would like to soak your beans ahead, this will shorten your cooking time. Put the beans in a large bowl and cover with several inches of water. Let soak for as long as you can. Overnight is optimal but even a few hours will hasten the cooking.

2. When ready to cook, drain the beans and place them along with the oil, 3 of the garlic cloves, the celery, and the onion in a large pot over medium-high heat. Bundle the rosemary, thyme, and bay leaf together, tie securely with kitchen twine, and throw it into the pot (or just throw the untied herbs into the pot, though you will have to fish them out later). Add the Parmesan rind, if using. Cover everything with water and stir in the salt. Bring to a boil,

[CONTINUED]

then reduce the heat to medium and allow it to simmer, partially covered, until the beans are soft. This can take anywhere from 1 to 3 hours, depending upon how long (if at all) you soaked your beans and how old your dried beans were when you got them.

A test of doneness is to place a bean in your palm and blow on it (the natural thing to do since it will be hot). If the skin breaks, it's ready. Of course, tasting it is a better way to tell. If your bean pot starts to look dry before the beans finish cooking, add more water as needed. At the end of cooking, the water should not quite cover the beans. (If it's too liquidy, ladle the extra out and discard.)

3. Meanwhile, while the beans are cooking, prepare the farro. In a large pot of boiling salted water, cook the farro, pasta style, until softened. This could take anywhere from 20 minutes to an hour, depending upon what kind you use (see What Else?). Drain well.

4. Mince the remaining 2 garlic cloves.

5. When the beans are cooked, remove and discard the onion, celery, herbs, and Parmesan rind if you used it (you can leave the garlic cloves in the pot; they are yummy). Ladle half of the beans into a food processor or blender, add the minced raw garlic, and puree. Return the bean puree to the pot. (You can skip this step and just stir in the minced garlic; the broth will be thinner but just as tasty).

6. Serve the beans in bowls over the farro, drizzle each portion with plenty of olive oil, then sprinkle with good flaky salt, red pepper, and celery leaves or parsley. If the stew tastes a bit flat, swirl in some lemon juice at the end to perk up the flavors. Grated Parmesan cheese on top is also nice. But make sure not to skimp on the oil, salt, and red pepper when serving. It really makes the whole thing come together.

What Else?

- A note about the beans. If you notice, soaking is purely optional here. I find that if I simmer them with enough water, they eventually cook up just fine without the soaking. And I'm the kind of person who usually doesn't plan tomorrow's dinner the evening before, which is ideally when you'd want to get those beans tucked into their bowl of water for the night. However, if you are a plan aheader, then go ahead and soak them. They will cook up faster if you do, which will save on fuel. Some people also say they find soaked beans more digestible. I haven't really noticed a big difference (code for beans don't really make me gassy, so why bother).

- Substitute any dried bean you like for the cannellini beans. This basic bean recipe will work with any of them, though the cooking times will vary.

- Look for semi-pearled farro. It cooks more quickly than whole farro—20 minutes instead of an hour.

- If you can't find farro, you can substitute wheat berries. These will take hours to cook, though, so leave yourself plenty of time. Or try brown rice or whole wheat Israeli couscous.

- If you are in a meaty mood, feel free to lard the pot with a ham hock or two, some bacon, a smoked turkey neck or wing, or some sautéed sausage. If you use meat, you definitely don't need the Parmesan rind (though it won't hurt).

- To turn this into a soup, add more water and salt to taste. Or use a good quality vegetable or chicken broth instead of half the water.

- To add some color and turn this into more of a whole meal, add a bunch or package of spinach, or a small bunch of kale (torn into pieces). Simmer until the greens wilt before serving.

TUSCAN KALE WITH ANCHOVIES, GARLIC, AND PECORINO

In the winter months, I come home from the farmers' market every week with at least two or three bunches of different braising greens, and I cook them all week long. That splash of chlorophyll always brightens my night and makes me feel happy and even sort of virtuous, regardless of whether I'm serving them with steamed fish or roasted pork belly.

Usually, I take the minimalist approach and just sauté the greens in olive oil with some garlic and a pinch or two of crushed red pepper flakes. But every once in a while, I'll gussy everything up with some anchovies and cheese to add tang and depth. This is the kind of recipe that you will most probably serve as a side dish (it's terrific with white beans and brilliant with roast pork of any description). But when I'm home alone, I'll halve the recipe and cook it up for my dinner, with some hot buttered toast or quick-cooking polenta. An egg, fried in olive oil until crisp brown around the edges but still runny-yolked, slid on top just before serving makes it even more substantially dinner-like. And a big glass of red wine never hurts.

Serves 4

2 bunches Tuscan kale
2 tablespoons olive oil
6 anchovy fillets
2 to 3 fat garlic cloves, finely chopped
Lots of freshly ground black pepper
2 ounces pecorino cheese, grated (about 1/2 cup), optional
Kosher or coarse sea salt, if needed

1. Remove the center ribs from the kale and discard; tear the leaves into bite-size pieces. Rinse well but do not dry (you want the moisture on the leaves to help steam them as they cook).
2. In a large skillet over medium heat, warm the oil. Stir in the anchovies and cook until dissolved, about 1 minute. Stir in the garlic and cook until slightly softened, about a minute.
3. Add the damp kale a handful at a time, letting each handful wilt slightly before adding more; toss well. Cook until the greens are completely wilted, about 5 minutes. If the kale is still tough but the pan is dry, splash in a little more water and let cook. For very tough greens you might need to repeat this. Season the kale with pepper and toss with cheese (if desired) and salt to taste before serving.

What Else?

- You can substitute almost any other braising green for the Tuscan kale (which is also called lacinato kale and dinosaur kale). Other kale varieties, Swiss chard, spinach, and mustard greens melt down into the pan beautifully as well. Collards will also work, but you need to slice them into thin ribbons so they cook quickly. If they are still tough after a few minutes over the heat, add 1/4 cup of water to the pan and let it cook off. They should be tender by then. If they seem especially leathery, you can blanch the collards first for a few minutes in lots of boiling water, then drain and add them to the skillet.

A Dish by Another Name

- Sautéed Kale with Hot Pepper and Cumin: Ditch the anchovies, cheese, and black pepper. Add a pinch of crushed red pepper flakes and a teaspoon of whole cumin seeds along with the garlic.

[CONTINUED]

- Wilted Kale with Garlic and Lemon: Ditch the anchovies. Toss the kale with a big squeeze of lemon juice before adding the cheese, if using.

- Practically Naked Kale: Only try this with really good, fresh kale. Ditch everything in the recipe save for the kale, oil, and salt. Sauté the kale in the oil and season with salt. This is really nice when you've got palate fatigue or are too darn tired to chop up a garlic clove.

CRISP ROASTED CHICKEN WITH CHICKPEAS, LEMONS, AND CARROTS WITH PARSLEY GREMOLATA

When I flip through food magazines, I rarely read the recipes. I look at the photos and imagine what I think the recipe *should* be. Most of the time I get it pretty close, but sometimes I'm way off base. This recipe is an example of that.

The photo was of a roasted chicken on a bed of chickpeas and what I thought were tiny cubes of carrot. I could taste the dish in my head. The chickpeas were crunchy and salty next to the melting, sweet carrots, and everything was suffused with chicken fat from the roasting bird.

In fact, the carrots turned out to be bits of orange bell pepper (definitely not in season in January in New York) and the chickpeas were added to the pan during the last few minutes of cooking so they would stay moist and soft, without the time to absorb much in the way of chicken essence. I'm sure it was a perfectly good dish, but I liked my own idea better.

So next time I roasted a chicken, I tried it.

I placed the chicken on a rack over the chickpeas and carrot slices so all the good juices would drip down onto them. I also added slivered lemon because I love the way lemons caramelize when you roast them, and I figured the dish would need some zip to perk up the garam masala, a spicy, earthy Indian spice blend I rubbed on the bird.

While it roasted, I chopped together a mix of parsley, lemon zest, and garlic known as gremolata (which is usually served with osso buco) to sprinkle on top. I knew it would give the whole thing some color and a little kick from the garlic, which would be welcome with all the hearty flavors.

When everything was done, the chicken was burnished, shining, and

[CONTINUED]

fragrant, the chickpeas, lemon bits, and carrots caramelized and tender. It was so pretty I immediately had to take a picture, which looks nothing like the food porn photo that was its inspiration. I can't say how the flavors compare, but my chicken was darned good—intensely lemony, very succulent, the chickpeas as tempting as bacon. Maybe one day I'll dig up that other recipe to give it a whirl . . . though given how delightful this dish is, maybe not.

Serves 4

FOR THE CHICKEN

2 lemons

2 (15-ounce) cans chickpeas, drained, or 3½ cups cooked chickpeas

2 tablespoons extra-virgin olive oil

1½ tablespoons garam masala

3 teaspoons kosher salt

1½ teaspoons freshly ground black pepper

1 (3½-pound) whole chicken, rinsed and patted dry

4 thyme sprigs

3 tablespoons unsalted butter, softened

1 pound carrots, peeled, trimmed, and cut into 1-inch rounds

FOR THE GREMOLATA

3 tablespoons chopped fresh parsley

½ teaspoon finely grated lemon zest

1 small garlic clove, finely chopped

1. Preheat the oven to 400°F. Quarter the lemons lengthwise and remove and discard any seeds. Thinly slice 6 of the lemon quarters crosswise (you will get little triangles) and in a bowl, toss them with the chickpeas, oil, ½ tablespoon (which equals 1½ teaspoons if you don't have a ½-tablespoon measure) garam masala, 1 teaspoon salt, and ½ teaspoon pepper.

2. Season the inside of the chicken cavity with 1 teaspoon salt and ½ teaspoon pepper. Fill the cavity with the remaining lemon wedges and thyme sprigs. Rub the outside of the chicken all over with the remaining 1 table-

16

COOK This NOW

spoon garam masala, 1 teaspoon salt, and $\frac{1}{2}$ teaspoon pepper. Rub the butter all over the skin.

3. Scatter the carrots in the bottom of the largest roasting pan you have (the one you use for your Thanksgiving turkey). Place a wire roasting rack over the carrots; arrange the chicken, breast-side up, on the rack. Transfer the pan to the oven and roast, stirring the carrots occasionally, for 30 minutes. Scatter the chickpea mixture into the bottom of the roasting pan. Continue to roast until the chicken's thigh juices run clear when pierced with a knife, 45 to 60 minutes longer. Let the chicken rest 5 minutes before carving.

4. Meanwhile, combine the parsley, lemon zest, and garlic in a bowl. Spoon the carrot-chickpea mixture onto a platter; arrange the chicken on top. Sprinkle the gremolata over the dish and serve.

What Else?

- Some farmers' market chickens have tough old legs because they develop actual muscle tone from the exercise they get pecking for grubs around the farm. If you suspect you've got one like this (or you know you do from prior experience with a particular farm), you might want to carve them off the chicken carcass and give them a head start in the oven before adding the breast. That way your breast won't dry out in the time that the legs will need to soften. To do this, carve the legs off the bird and smear those legs and the rest of the chicken carcass with the butter, salt, and seasonings. Put the legs in the pan (along with the carrots) to roast for 15 minutes before adding the carcass with the breasts (tuck the lemon and herbs inside the cavity before roasting). The overall time will be a tad longer than called for above, so just keep checking to see when the juices run clear with a knife.

- Yes, you can eat the lemon, and it's delicious (in case you were wondering).

A Dish by Another Name

• For a more traditional Sunday Supper Roasted Chicken, you can skip the chickpeas and lemon bits and instead just add a pound of cubed potatoes to the pan along with the carrots. Season the carrots and potatoes with salt and pepper and give them a stir once or twice while the chicken roasts. This is good with or without the gremolata.

WHATEVER GREENS
YOU'VE GOT SALAD

No dinner at our house is complete without a salad, which we eat French style, after the entrée, usually on the same plate to soak up the last of any lingering juices. I'm a big fan of making a garlic mustard vinaigrette when I have time, but usually the dressing gets short shrift since tossing the greens with vinegar and oil right in the bowl takes about 12 seconds. On a weeknight I often don't have the 3 minutes it takes to paste the garlic clove.

I'll say this for garlic and mustard dressings, though: When I do take the time to make it, even my toddler, Dahlia, will put a leaf or two in her mouth. Usually she just licks off the vinaigrette, but occasionally she will swallow the lettuce. And in summer, I'll let her rifle through the bowl and pull out the cucumbers (I know, indulgent—but I figure any way to get her to eat her veggies is okay with me).

Daniel always knows I'm in a very bad way—either emotionally or physically—when I leave the salad untouched on my plate. That's when he makes me a toddy and puts me to bed. This is a highly rare occurrence because I really do love salad.

Serves 4

2 quarts salad greens (use whatever you've got), washed and spun dry
Large pinch kosher or sea salt
1 teaspoon vinegar, any kind you like, more to taste
Good olive oil to taste

1. Pile the lettuce leaves in a big salad bowl. Ideally your bowl should be filled only about two-thirds full with greens so you have room to toss.
2. In a tiny bowl, mix the salt with the vinegar. This dissolves the salt. Pour it on your greens and toss well. Taste a leaf. If it's salty and tart enough, dribble in the oil and toss well until combined. (If not, add more salt and

[CONTINUED]

vinegar; the exact amount will depend on the acid level of the vinegar you use: The more tart it is, the less you need.) The best way to toss the salad is with your hands. You'll be able to feel when the salad is perfectly coated with dressing, which is harder to do when you and the greens are separated by salad tossers or tongs. Rooting around with all that oil in the bowl is nicely emollient for your hands, too—always a plus. Serve at once.

What Else?

- In winter, my go-to salad green is spinach because that's what I can get at the farmers' market on a regular basis. It makes a hearty, mineral-tasting salad with a deep green flavor. But use whatever you've got.

- The choices in both oil and vinegar are myriad here. Simply change the vinegar or the type of oil and the whole character of the salad will change. Olive oil is my standard but don't forget about nut oils if you've got them stashed in the fridge: hazelnut or walnut. This winter I've fallen in love with pumpkin seed and squash seed oils, which have a fruity, forest-like flavor with a nutty nuance. For a gentle flavor, grapeseed oil is sweetly mellow. The vinegars in my pantry are numerous as well, including sherry vinegar, red and white wine vinegars, balsamic, rice wine (mild and lovely with butter lettuce and cucumbers), cider vinegar, and malt vinegar—which I actually never use for green salads (it's strong, but good in a potato salad). Some of my favorite oil/vinegar combinations are nut oils with sherry vinegar, pumpkin seed oil with balsamic, and olive oil with red or white wine vinegar (an oldie but a goody).

- When my dairy-avoiding husband Daniel isn't around, I generally add cheese to salad, everything from a sprinkle of grated Parmesan to crumbled feta or goat cheese, grated Gruyère, or cubed pecorino. I love the slight bit of richness next to the crisp, cold greens.

- If you are a lemon lover, and I most certainly am, substitute fresh lemon juice for the vinegar.

A Dish by Another Name

- To make Mustard and Garlic Vinaigrette, paste up a garlic clove with a pinch of salt (you can use a mortar and pestle or a knife). Put it in a small bowl with another pinch of salt, a dab of mustard (maybe $1/2$ teaspoon), a few drops of vinegar, and a minced anchovy if you like. Mix well with a fork or whisk, then slowly mix in the olive oil until it tastes good. Then stop. Leave it on the strong side because once it's tossed with the greens, the flavor becomes diluted. You can always add more oil after it's tossed with the salad if it is still too strong, but if you make it too wimpy to start, it's harder to fix. (For a more specific recipe, see page 41.)

SESAME SOBA SALAD WITH ROASTED SHIITAKES AND TOFU CROUTONS

For most of my life, I ate buckwheat one way—as kasha at my grandmother's table. She served it in the traditional Russian Jewish style, boiled until just shy of mushy, then topped with sweet, charred, near-black onions and plenty of sautéed mushrooms on top.

Then I went to college and discovered a whole other buckwheat culture bobbing away in the soup pots of the Upper West Side's Japanese restaurants. Smooth, gentle soba noodles immediately replaced nubby kasha as my favorite buckwheat endeavor and they still are. I just love how the smoky earthiness of the grain is softened by the noodles' silky, slippery texture, which slide past my lips when slicked with broth or oil (in this case fragrant, toasty sesame oil).

This robust and sustaining soba salad, seasoned with ginger, orange juice, and soy sauce and garnished with crunchy cucumber, is an ideal dish to serve to all your gluten-free vegetarian friends, of which I have at least one, on Twitter anyway. Just make sure you buy certified gluten-free soba noodles because although pure buckwheat is naturally gluten-free (despite the name, buckwheat is a grass and not a grain), soba noodles are sometimes made with regular wheat flour.

FOR THE SALAD

Serves 4

7 to 8 ounces shiitake mushrooms, stems removed

2 tablespoons toasted (Asian) sesame oil, more to taste

3 1/2 tablespoons soy sauce, more to taste

Pinch kosher salt

1/2 (12.8-ounce) package soba noodles

1 1/2 tablespoons freshly squeezed orange juice (about half a small orange)

1 tablespoon rice wine vinegar

1 tablespoon grated gingerroot

COOK *This* NOW

1 medium cucumber, peeled

2 scallions, thinly sliced

2 tablespoons chopped fresh cilantro

1 tablespoon lightly toasted sesame seeds

FOR THE CROUTONS (OPTIONAL, SEE WHAT ELSE?)

½ pound extra-firm tofu, drained and sliced into ¾-inch slabs

1 tablespoon peanut or olive oil

2 tablespoons tamari or soy sauce

1½ teaspoons toasted (Asian) sesame oil

1. Preheat the oven to 400°F. Slice the mushroom caps into ¼-inch strips. Toss the mushrooms with 1 tablespoon sesame oil, ½ tablespoon soy sauce, and a pinch of salt. Spread the mushrooms out in a single layer on a baking sheet. Roast, tossing occasionally, until the mushrooms are tender and slightly golden, 8 to 10 minutes.

2. Cook the soba noodles according to the package instructions. Drain and rinse quickly under cold running water; drain again completely.

3. In a bowl, whisk together the remaining 3 tablespoons soy sauce and 1 tablespoon sesame oil, the orange juice, vinegar, and ginger.

4. Cut the cucumber lengthwise into quarters and scoop out the seeds with a spoon. Cut each quarter crosswise into thin slices.

5. To prepare the tofu croutons, pat the tofu slabs dry with a paper towel. Heat the oil in a nonstick pan. When it shimmers, add the tofu and let it cook undisturbed (stand away from the tofu) for 3 minutes. It should be golden brown on the bottom. Flip the tofu pieces and continue to cook for about 2 minutes longer, until the underside is golden. In a small bowl, whisk together the tamari or soy sauce and sesame oil. Pour it in the pan with the croutons and cook for 1 minute longer. Drain croutons on a paper towel–lined plate.

6. In a large bowl, toss together the noodles, cucumber, mushrooms, scallions, cilantro, sesame seeds, and dressing. Serve topped with tofu croutons, if desired. Drizzle the salad with more soy sauce and sesame oil just before serving if it needs perking up.

What Else?

- If you don't feel like frying up the tofu, you can leave it out, though you will miss its crunch against all the soft noodles. Plain cubes of raw tofu are also a nice, pillowy addition. Toss them with a little sesame oil and soy sauce and then scatter them over the noodles before serving.

- To be more seasonal about this salad, omit the cucumber. Radishes or sweet raw turnips (especially the tiny Japanese ones called haruki), sliced thinly, will work really well as a substitute, and I toyed with the idea of listing them instead of the cucumber in the recipe itself. But when it comes down to it, I always use cucumber because I like its juiciness. So, in the name of honesty, I'm telling it like it is.

- If you are not a tofu fan or just in the mood for a variation, top the salad with sautéed shrimp or scallops instead. Soft little bay scallops fried in sesame oil with a sprinkle of flaky, crunchy salt would be fabulous.

- If you like spicy, garnish the salad with a squirt of Sriracha or other hot sauce. This is how Daniel eats it.

PORT WINE–BRAISED OXTAILS (OR SHORT RIBS)

I had eaten oxtails, mostly in terrines, many times over the years in fancy French restaurants, and enjoyed them well enough in a meaty, brisket-like way. But I didn't fall head over heels until I had them still on the bone, stewed Southern style, at Sylvia's up in Harlem.

I was working on a cookbook with the estimable Sylvia Woods, the proprietress, and every evening when we'd finish our interviewing, she'd send me home to Brooklyn with dinner. I'd spend the hour-long subway ride balancing warm take-out containers of fragrant food on my lap, my stomach growling. My then husband and I would devour them minutes after I walked in the door: macaroni and cheese, fried chicken, collard greens with bits of smoked turkey, and oxtails, still on the bone in a thin brown gravy. To eat them, I used my fingers and sucked the meat right off, along with marrow from the twisty crevices. Then I'd gnaw away at any tendons still clinging. It was all so soft and rich and fatty and full flavored, I was instantly hooked.

The thing is, oxtails are not the kind of dish I make at home on a regular basis. They are hard to find, and not necessarily to everyone's liking. Plus, because of the inelegant, gnawing, chomping way that I like to eat them, it's not a dish I'm going to tuck into in front of most company.

But when my dear friend Ana from Vashon Island, Washington, decided to come and visit last January, I knew that she would not only tolerate my—let's say, enthusiastic—oxtail table manners, she'd actually applaud them.

I was able to procure the meat from the farmers' market by putting in an order with a meat farmer well in advance. Most butchers do carry them if you inquire. They usually come frozen and need a day's thawing in the fridge. Oxtail is not a spur-of-the-moment kind of thing.

Instead of making oxtails à la Sylvia in a simple gravy, I decided to doll them up a bit and braise them as I do short ribs, in a reduction of red wine and

[CONTINUED]

port. This made them a little sweet and very complex tasting, with a shiny, full-bodied sauce (if you aren't an oxtail fan, you can make this same recipe with short ribs—see What Else?). The house smelled meaty and winey and utterly divine all afternoon as they simmered. And they glistened invitingly when mounded on a platter with roasted potatoes and turnips.

After a few minutes of attempting fork and knife, both Ana and Daniel abandoned their cutlery and joined my fingerful feast. It was a bit of work to get at the good meat, but, like crabs and lobster, it's entirely worth it.

1 (750-ml) bottle dry red wine

½ cup ruby port

4½ pounds large oxtail pieces, rinsed and patted dry

Kosher salt, for seasoning

Freshly ground black pepper, for seasoning

2 tablespoons unsalted butter

1 tablespoon olive oil

5 shallots, finely chopped

5 garlic cloves, finely chopped

2 medium leeks, chopped

1 celery stalk, finely chopped

3 thyme sprigs

2 rosemary sprigs

1 bunch parsley stems (use some of the leaves for garnish, if you like)

2 bay leaves

2 medium carrots, scrubbed and diced small

Balsamic vinegar to taste

Serves 4

1. Preheat the oven to 325°F. In a large saucepan over high heat, bring the wine and port to a boil. Lower the heat and simmer until reduced by half, about 20 minutes.

2. Meanwhile, brown the oxtails. Season them generously with salt and pepper (you will need at least 2 teaspoons salt and a teaspoon pepper, or even more if it feels right). In a large Dutch oven over medium-high heat, melt

1 tablespoon of the butter with the olive oil. Working in batches, arrange the oxtails in a single layer and brown on all sides. Take your time with this and let them get good and brown; don't crowd the pan, or they will steam and never develop that tasty caramelized crust. Transfer the oxtails to a bowl.

3. Melt the remaining tablespoon of butter in the Dutch oven and add the shallots, garlic, leeks, and celery. Cook the vegetables, scraping up the browned bits on the bottom of the pan, until softened, stirring constantly, about 5 minutes.

4. Arrange the oxtails over the vegetables and add the reduced wine-port mixture. Using kitchen twine, tie together the thyme, rosemary, parsley stems, and bay leaves, and drop into the pot. (You can skip the twine and simply drop the herbs in the pot; it will be a more rustic presentation but rare is the guest who will call you out on it. Besides, these are *oxtails*; they are not supposed to be fancy in a short ribs way.) Bring the liquid to a boil on the stovetop, then cover and transfer the Dutch oven to the oven. Cook, turning the oxtails occasionally, until the meat is tender but not yet falling off the bone, 2 to 2$1/2$ hours. Add the carrots and let cook for another 30 minutes.

5. If you're serving the stew right away, you can try to spoon off some of the fat from the surface if it looks a little greasy. Or chill the stew overnight so the fat hardens and then it will be simple to take off. Reheat if necessary, then season with balsamic vinegar and additional salt, if desired. Serve the oxtails in a bowl topped with parsley leaves if you need to break up all the brown.

What Else?

- If you are a mashed potato kind of person (and really, other than my unfathomable toddler, who isn't?), serve these over mashed potatoes. You won't regret it.

A Dish by Another Name

- Port Wine–Braised Short Ribs: Substitute 3 pounds short ribs for the oxtails. Flanken, which are short ribs cut across the bone (and which are, for some reason, cheaper than traditional short ribs), also work. So will plain old beef stew meat; use 2 pounds boneless meat.

- Port Wine–Braised Lamb Shanks: Substitute 4 lamb foreshanks.

- Port Wine–Braised Pot Roast: Substitute 2 to 3 pounds brisket or chuck roast.

SKILLET-ROASTED POTATOES AND GOLDEN TURNIPS WITH SMASHED GARLIC

For years, I didn't cook with turnips nearly enough, usually casting them aside for denser, sweeter roots such as parsnips, rutabagas, and carrots. But at the market this winter I discovered golden turnips, a particularly mellow variety with a pretty yellow color. Like all root vegetables, if you roast them, they will caramelize and condense into something honeyed and browned. I've also boiled and mashed them with lots of butter, and they're quite wonderful—lighter than mashed potatoes and more intensely flavored, too, with their distinctive turnip-y tang.

If you are unsure about whether or not you like turnips, try this recipe, which pairs them in equal parts with Yukon Gold potatoes, seasoned with garlic and bay leaf. Once, I cooked them in the same oven as a pot of port-braised oxtails (page 25), and they went terrifically well together.

Serves 4

1 pound Yukon Gold potatoes, cut into 3/4-inch cubes
1 pound golden turnips, peeled and cut into 3/4-inch cubes
2 1/2 tablespoons extra-virgin olive oil
1 teaspoon kosher or coarse sea salt
1/2 teaspoon freshly ground black pepper
3 unpeeled garlic cloves, smashed
2 bay leaves

1. Preheat the oven to 325°F. In a large cast-iron or other oven-safe skillet, toss together all of the ingredients.

2. Transfer the skillet to the oven and cook, mixing every 20 minutes, until the vegetables are golden and tender, about 1 1/2 hours. If you want them even more crusty and browned, run the pan under the broiler for a few

[CONTINUED]

minutes to sear the surface. This is entirely optional; they are terrific without the extra color.

What Else?

- You can use regular turnips or baby turnips in place of the golden turnips. Ditto rutabaga cubes or carrot chunks. Or try this recipe with just potatoes— it's a great way to cook them.

- If you have thyme sprigs and prefer them to bay leaves, swap them out.

BAKED APPLES WITH FIG AND CARDAMOM CRUMBLE

Here's what I love about apple crumble: the crumbly, nubby, cinnamon-sweet topping. Here's what I don't love about apple crumble: the mushy, applesauce-like fruit at the bottom.

This recipe fixes the mush factor without compromising the crumbly bits on top. My trick is to quarter rather than slice the apples. The larger pieces won't break down as quickly or as much, but they do soften to a luscious spoonable-ness. Bigger apple pieces also make the dish easier and faster to put together.

The last time I made apple crumble, I also threw in some dried figs plumped in brandy to give the dish pockets of sweet, chewy goodness. Feel free to leave them out if you don't like dried figs. Or substitute a dried fruit that you do like. Dried apricot slices, cherries, and cranberries would be marvelous and very pretty.

Serves 6 to 8

FOR THE FRUIT

3 tablespoons brandy

1 cup dried figs, roughly chopped

4 large apples (about 3 pounds), peeled, cored, and quartered

2 tablespoons granulated sugar

2 teaspoons freshly squeezed lemon juice

$1/2$ teaspoon ground cardamom

2 tablespoons unsalted butter, melted

FOR THE CRUMBLE TOPPING

$1/2$ cup all-purpose flour

$1/4$ cup plus 3 tablespoons light brown sugar

$1/4$ cup whole wheat flour

$1/4$ cup rolled oats

[CONTINUED]

3/4 teaspoon ground cardamom
1/2 teaspoon ground ginger
1/8 teaspoon kosher salt
3/4 cup (1 1/2 sticks) unsalted butter, cold and cut into pieces
Crème fraîche or Greek yogurt, for serving

1. Preheat the oven to 375°F. Lightly grease a 9 × 9-inch square baking pan.
2. In a small saucepan, bring the brandy to a simmer. Take it off the heat, add the chopped figs, and cover the pan. Allow the figs to plump in the liquid for 30 minutes.
3. To prepare the crumble, in a bowl, mix together the all-purpose flour, brown sugar, whole wheat flour, oats, cardamom, ginger, and salt. Add the butter pieces and mix in with your fingers or a fork until large crumbs form.
4. For the apples, in a large bowl, toss the apples with the granulated sugar, lemon juice, and cardamom. Add the melted butter and toss again until the apples are coated. Stir in the figs along with any unabsorbed brandy.
5. Scrape the apple mixture into the prepared pan and top with an even layer of the crumble. Bake until the apples are tender and the topping is golden brown, 45 to 50 minutes. Transfer the pan to a wire rack to cool slightly, 15 to 20 minutes. Serve warm if you can, with a dollop of crème fraîche or Greek yogurt.

What Else?

-   You can use any apple varieties here. A mix of apples works well because then you get a range of textures and flavors. When choosing apples, remember that dense, crisp apples will yield firmer, more intact apple chunks while softer apples break down and turn a little saucy. Both types are good, just different.

-   This homey dessert loves creamy company—any type will do. I serve it to Dahlia dribbled with heavy cream. Once, when I didn't have any yogurt or cream in the house (a rare and dreadful occurrence), I ate a bowl topped with some ricotta (yum). Ice cream, especially a slightly exotic flavor such as ginger or green tea, would make this dinner-party suitable.

- This makes a fine brunch or breakfast dish if you skew the ratio of apple crumble to yogurt in favor of the yogurt. It's sort of like a bowl of fruit and granola, but with baked apples instead of fresh berries and bananas and the like.

- You can use all whole wheat flour for the topping. It's a tad heavier but really not by that much. I slightly prefer the mix of flours, but half the time when I make this I just use all whole wheat and no one can really tell the difference, especially when I serve it with ice cream (see above).

- If you are an absolute crumble topping lover, you can double the crumb part of the recipe. You might have to bake it for a few extra minutes to make sure it crisps through.

- If you love salty sweet desserts, try serving this with some thin slices of Cheddar or other firm cheese (young pecorino would be nice). Chunks of ricotta salata would also be lovely and unexpected.

MALLOBARS

This is my version of homemade Mallomars. But instead of painstakingly forming individual cookies, I use the bar cookie method, spreading everything in one large pan. I end up with a crisp, homemade graham cracker crust topped by honey marshmallow and a thick layer of chocolate. Though they are easier than the original recipe, I wouldn't call them a super-quick dessert. You still need to devote a good part of an afternoon to their confection. Or try to make the components over several days if it's easier to carve that out of your schedule.

However you manage it, the payoff is big: They are truly scrumptious, and I guarantee that if you bring them to a potluck or party, no one else will have brought anything remotely like them. They are unusual, crowd pleasing, fancy looking, and even slightly good for you (okay, just slightly) from the whole wheat flour.

FOR THE GRAHAM CRACKER BASE

1 cup (2 sticks) unsalted butter

1/4 cup firmly packed dark brown sugar

1/4 cup granulated sugar

1/4 cup honey

1 1/2 cups whole wheat flour

1 cup all-purpose flour

1 teaspoon kosher salt

1/2 teaspoon ground cinnamon

FOR THE HONEY MARSHMALLOW

3 envelopes unflavored gelatin (about 3 tablespoons)

1 cup cold water

2 cups granulated sugar

1/4 cup honey

2 large egg whites

Makes about 18
(2-inch) squares

1/4 teaspoon kosher salt

1 tablespoon vanilla extract

FOR THE CHOCOLATE GLAZE

9 ounces bittersweet chocolate, chopped

3/4 cup heavy cream

1. First, make the graham cracker base. In the bowl of an electric mixer, cream the butter, sugars, and honey until smooth. In a medium bowl, combine the flours, salt, and cinnamon. Add the dry ingredients to the mixer and beat until the dough just comes together.

2. Wrap the dough in plastic and pat into a disc. Chill the dough for at least 1 hour and up to 2 days.

3. When ready to bake, preheat the oven to 325°F. Line a 9 × 13-inch baking pan with foil or parchment paper. On a lightly floured surface, or in between two sheets of parchment paper, roll out the dough into a rectangle that just fits the prepared pan. Carefully transfer the dough to the prepared pan. Squish it to fit if it starts to tear (the dough is soft). Prick dough all over with a fork. Bake the graham cracker base until golden brown, 18 to 20 minutes. Allow the crust to cool completely before topping with the marshmallow. (The graham cracker base can be made a few days ahead; store, covered in foil, at room temperature.)

4. While the graham cracker base cools, prepare the honey marshmallow. Place the gelatin in the cold water to bloom. In a saucepan over medium heat, cook the sugar, honey, and 1/2 cup water, stirring until the sugar dissolves, until the mixture reaches 240°F on a candy thermometer.

5. In the bowl of an electric mixer, whisk the egg whites and salt until soft peaks form. When the sugar mixture has come up to temperature, carefully pour it into the egg whites while whisking. Continue whisking until the mixture has cooled slightly, about 1 minute, and add the gelatin and water mixture and the vanilla. Continue whisking until the mixture begins to thicken and quadruples in volume, 5 to 7 minutes. Scrape the marshmallow onto the graham cracker base and smooth the top with a spatula.

[CONTINUED]

Allow the marshmallow to set for 4 hours or overnight at room temperature.

6. To prepare the chocolate glaze, place the chocolate pieces in a bowl. In a saucepan over medium-high heat, bring the cream just to a boil. Pour the cream over the chocolate and whisk until the chocolate has melted and the glaze is smooth and shiny. Pour the glaze onto the set marshmallow and smooth with a spatula. Allow the glaze to set, about 30 minutes, before cutting into squares.

What Else?

• What else can I tell you? If these seem like too much trouble, you can always just go out and buy some Mallomars. And, being a seasonal product themselves (they are only available in the colder months), they arguably fit into a seasonal kitchen if you don't think about it all too deeply.

• The graham cracker dough also makes fantastic cookies all by itself. Just bake as directed above, but as soon as you take the pan out of the oven, while still hot, score the dough into 2-inch squares. Cool and break up into cookies.

DOUBLE COCONUT GRANOLA

"Granola is really oatmeal cookies in disguise," my friend Robin always says.

I know exactly what she means. Granola is addictive in the same, hard-to-stop-eating way as cookies, and when I have either in the house, I am completely and utterly at their mercy. Therefore, whenever I whip up a big batch of homemade granola, I only stash a little of it in the cupboard. The rest I pack up tightly in a jar and immediately hand off to Daniel so he can bring it to work (and far away from me). Otherwise, I am liable to scarf it down by the fistful and regret it later.

That said, if you can exercise more self-control, a batch of this is a good thing to keep in the pantry. It's very similar to an olive oil granola recipe I published in the *New York Times* (and in my last cookbook) with one major change. In place of the olive oil, I use virgin coconut oil (see What Else?). It makes for particularly crunchy oats with a deep coconut flavor that I play up by adding plenty of coconut chips to the mix. And virgin coconut oil is filled with lauric acid, which is also found in breast milk (you learn the darnedest things on the Internet), and which some research has shown both boosts the immune system and helps fight acne—though I suppose the acne part is for topical application. Not something you're likely to do with granola, no matter how addictive it is.

Makes about 7 cups

3 cups old-fashioned rolled oats

1½ cups coarsely chopped raw pecans

1 cup hulled raw pumpkin seeds

1 cup coconut chips

½ cup pure maple syrup

½ cup virgin coconut oil, melted

⅓ cup packed light brown sugar

1 teaspoon kosher salt

½ teaspoon ground cinnamon

[CONTINUED]

¼ teaspoon freshly grated nutmeg

¾ cup dried cherries

1. Preheat the oven to 300°F.
2. In a large bowl, combine the oats, pecans, pumpkin seeds, coconut chips, maple syrup, coconut oil, brown sugar, salt, cinnamon, and nutmeg. Spread the mixture on a rimmed baking sheet in an even layer and bake until golden all over, about 45 minutes, stirring every 10 minutes.
3. Transfer the granola to a large bowl and add the cherries, tossing to combine.

What Else?

- Virgin coconut oil is expensive, and if you don't want to spend the money or if you can't find it, you can substitute olive oil, which will pretty much give you a recipe similar to the olive oil granola originally published in the *Times*. I changed up the spices and dried fruit and nuts here to match the coconut oil, but they go nicely with olive oil as well. Melted butter is another possibility; it makes for a very rich granola with a slightly softer texture.

- As with any granola recipe, you can vary the fruits and nuts to suit yourself. Just make sure the dried fruit you use is nice and soft and plump.

- Homemade granola makes an amazing gift when it's packed into a pretty jar. Don't forget to attach a card with the recipe because I assure you, whoever you give it to will ask!

FEBRUARY

GRILLED SAUSAGES WITH CELERY ROOT SALAD WITH HAZELNUTS AND ARUGULA

During my junior year abroad in Paris, in between gobbling warm croissants, raw milk cheeses, and countless macaroons, I ate an awful lot of celery root rémoulade.

The mild, soft celery root, shaved into ribbons and cloaked in creamy mustard-spiked mayonnaise, appeared on every vegetable crudité platter I munched when I wanted a light lunch. I ate it slathered on pieces of crackle-crusted baguette, a small glass of rosé wine on the side. Abstemious it wasn't, but it was rich in vegetable matter, which, given the butter-chocolate-and-pâté reality of most of my diet, counted as moderation. And the colorful mélange of marinated beets, grated carrots, lettuce, corn, and pale celery root was just as beautiful to contemplate as to eat.

I never bothered making celery root rémoulade when I was in Paris because it was ubiquitous and cheap. Everyone, from the corner café to the fanciest traiteur, carried it. But once I got back to New York, if I wanted any more of that silky, savory salad, I'd have to tackle the homely root and whip some up myself.

And that's the thing about celery root rémoulade. It starts with celery roots, which, with their hairy skins and muddy crevices, are never going to be the most inviting vegetable in the bin. But once those roots are peeled and grated, a quick toss with lemony, mustard-imbued mayonnaise will make the most of their inner beauty.

These days, my celery root salad of choice is a lighter take on a rémoulade. Instead of mayonnaise, I use a zippy mustard vinaigrette, and serve the salad on a bed of tangy arugula topped with hazelnuts for crunch. It's marvelous as a first course on its own. Or to make it mealworthy, grill up your favorite sausages—lamb sausages are particularly good—and serve them alongside the salad, letting the mustard from the vinaigrette sauce the sausages and the sausage grease flavor the salad. And even though I'm no longer in Paris, a macaroon for dessert would not seem at all out of place.

FOR THE MUSTARD VINAIGRETTE
1 small garlic clove, finely chopped
1/4 teaspoon kosher salt plus 1 small pinch
1 teaspoon Dijon mustard
2 teaspoons sherry vinegar
3 tablespoons extra-virgin olive oil
Freshly ground black pepper to taste

1 1/4 pounds sausages, whatever kind you like

FOR THE SALAD
1 medium celery root, trimmed and peeled (see What Else?)
5 cups arugula or other salad green, torn into bite-size pieces
1/4 cup finely chopped toasted hazelnuts

1. To make the mustard vinaigrette, with a mortar and pestle or using the flat side of a knife, smash the garlic and tiny pinch of salt to make a paste. Whisk it in a small bowl with the mustard, vinegar, and remaining salt. Whisking constantly, slowly drizzle in the oil until fully incorporated. Season with pepper.

2. Preheat the broiler. Prick the sausages all over with a fork, then lay them on a baking sheet. Broil them about 3 inches from the heat until browned on both sides, 3 to 4 minutes per side (exactly how long will depend on your oven and the thickness of your sausage).

3. Fit a food processor with a large grating blade; grate the celery root. You can also use a box grater, though beware your knuckles. Transfer to a large bowl and add the salad greens and hazelnuts. Pour the vinaigrette over the salad and toss well. Season with more salt, lemon juice, and/or olive oil if needed before serving.

What Else?

- This recipe calls for a medium celery root, which is about the same size as a large navel orange (4 or 5 inches in diameter). If you can only get one of the giant, grapefruit-size roots, use about three-quarters of it. Or use it all; just make a little extra vinaigrette to make sure it's well seasoned.

- Trimming the celery root is probably the hardest and most annoying thing about this recipe. You can use a sharp vegetable peeler, but a sharp paring knife is more efficient. Either way, be prepared to go deep. You will likely need to hack off about a quarter inch of the surface to get past the divots of dirt.

- This goes really well with mashed Yukon Gold potatoes. To make them, try this: Boil the potatoes (unpeeled) in plenty of water until very soft. Drain, let cool, then slip off the skins. In the same pot you used to boil the potatoes, heat some milk or chicken stock seasoned with salt until simmering. Add the potatoes and a lump of butter (use as much as you can bear; my tolerance is high), and mash with a potato masher or fork over very low heat until as smooth as you like it. We like lumps. Sometimes I leave the skin on the potatoes. Serve at once.

CRISPY BROWN BUTTER MUSHROOMS

My daughter, Dahlia, won't touch potatoes (sweet potatoes included), spits out roasted butternut squash, and says "no thank you" to carrots, but she absolutely loves mushrooms. Broiled in olive oil or fried in butter, as long as they are crisp edged, hot, and sprinkled with salt, she'll devour as many as I put on her plate—without me having to resort to my usual "but Elmo *loves* mushrooms" tactics.

So I make them often. But I discovered by accident how good they are with brown butter. One frantic dinnertime while I simultaneously sliced pineapple and boiled up whole wheat macaroni, I forgot about the butter melting in the skillet for the mushrooms. The nutty, caramelized, milky scent wafting around the kitchen reminded me, and by the time I looked at the pan, the butter was golden and fragrant but luckily not burned. With the clock ticking I threw in the mushrooms, and good things happened as they cooked and crisped. The brown butter added a sweet, nutty richness that went perfectly with the mushrooms' funky, woodsy flavor.

Still, you can easily make this recipe with olive oil instead of butter. One year at my annual Hanukkah latkes party, I did just that, frying them up and serving them in a crinkly mound sprinkled with salt. They went even faster than the latkes, though they did have novelty on their side.

Serves 4 as a side dish or first course

1 pound mushrooms, preferably maitake if you can get them
    (also called hen-of-the-woods mushrooms); oyster mushrooms
    work well, too
4 tablespoons butter or olive oil
Few drops fresh lemon juice, if you like
Flaky sea salt to taste

[CONTINUED]

1. Give the mushrooms a very quick rinse, then shake dry. Trim into ½-inch pieces.

2. In your largest skillet over medium heat, melt the butter. The skillet should be large enough for all the mushrooms to fit in one layer without crowding. If it's smaller, cook the mushrooms in batches, because if you crowd them, they will steam and turn soggy instead of becoming brown and crisp.

3. When the foam has subsided from the butter, let the butter continue to cook until it smells nutty and you start to see light brown specks on the bottom. This is a very light brown butter, which will darken further after you add the mushrooms. Add the mushrooms. Let them cook without moving them until their bottoms are deeply golden brown, about 3 minutes. Flip the mushrooms and let them cook on their other side until crisp, about 3 minutes longer. Season with lemon juice, if you like, and plenty of sea salt, and serve hot hot hot.

What Else?

- Some people say that if you wash your mushrooms, they will absorb too much water and become soggy and bloated. This might be true with a long soak, but with a quick rinse under a gentle faucet, I've never noticed a difference. If you'd rather not subject your mushrooms to any kind of dunking, you can rub them down with a damp paper towel.

- If you can't get maitake mushrooms, substitute the most interesting kind of mushroom you can get (except for shiitakes, which turn leathery here). In a pinch even white button mushrooms will taste great prepared this way. Just slice them up and fry as directed. You might have to adjust the cooking time slightly depending on the variety you use; just watch the mushrooms carefully so they don't burn.

- If you are using maitake mushrooms, this recipe truly needs nothing else. It's one of those minimalist marvels that transcends its basic ingredients. However, if you're into lily gilding, here are some ideas for embellishments:

- Garnish with toasted pine nuts or toasted slivered almonds.
- Dust with chopped chives before serving.
- Drizzle with a tiny touch of good balsamic vinegar.
- Shower with freshly grated Parmesan while the mushrooms are still in the pan, then toss until the cheese melts.

- Leftover mushrooms are excellent with scrambled eggs. Or add them to sautéed onions to make into a frittata. Even a few tablespoons of these mushrooms, finely chopped, will add a lot of flavor wherever you add them. Once, I added them to pasta sauce, not enough for anyone to notice, but just enough to deepen the taste of everything else, thanks to the mushrooms' umami factor.

- You can serve these as a side dish with almost anything—fish, meats, pasta, eggs. Or toss them into a salad to turn everyday salad greens into something dinner party–worthy and elegant.

CHILE-COCONUT BRAISED
BEEF SHORT RIBS

When Dahlia turned one, Daniel and I decided we wanted to have professional pictures taken of our little family. So I asked our friend and neighbor Lucy Schaeffer if she'd be interested in trading a family photo session for a catered dinner made by me.

Lucy is one of the most talented food photographers out there. She's worked on many cookbooks, but she also has a special interest in photographing children and is brilliant at it. She knew just what to do to get our then twelve-month-old to smile and coo on cue (if only she could move in with us and do this all the time).

We spent a lovely fall afternoon taking photos in the garden, and in exchange I delivered a home-cooked dinner to her family. This chile-flecked, creamy, slow-cooked beef dish is what she chose out of a long list of entrée possibilities.

Now, here is a confession. When I sent her the entrée ideas, I'd never made any of them before. I just sat around and dreamed up the most tempting and delicious-sounding dishes I could fathom. I chose braised meats as a focus, since they are easy to make in advance and deliver to your neighbor's door without losing anything in the journey.

I knew I wanted the beef to be very succulent, so I bought boneless short ribs and cut them into large cubes. As they cooked in a mixture of coconut milk, chiles, and spices, the whole house filled with rich and meaty aromas and Daniel started asking me when dinner would be ready. Sadly, I had to tell him that we were eating pasta. The beef was for Lucy's family.

When it was ready, Daniel and I stole a few pieces of meat before forcing ourselves to pack up the rest of it. Then I made the dish all over again the very next day. The second batch tasted even better to us, though anticipation might have had something to do with that.

Serves 6

2 pounds boneless beef short ribs, cut into 2-inch chunks

1½ teaspoons kosher salt, more to taste

1 teaspoon chili powder (you can use hot or mild)

½ teaspoon freshly ground black pepper, more to taste

1 tablespoon coconut oil or olive oil, for searing

4 garlic cloves, minced

2 jalapeños, deveined and deseeded, if desired, and minced

2 inches fresh ginger, grated

1 small shallot, minced

½ teaspoon cumin seeds

1 (13.5-ounce) can coconut milk

Freshly squeezed juice and finely grated zest of 2 limes, plus additional wedges for serving, if desired

Chopped cilantro, for serving

Chopped scallions, for serving

1. Preheat the oven to 325°F. Season the beef all over with a teaspoon of the salt, the chili powder, and black pepper. In a 5-quart Dutch oven over medium-high heat, heat the oil. Add the beef and cook until browned all over, about 8 minutes. Add the garlic, jalapeños, ginger, shallot, and cumin seeds and cook, stirring, until everything is fragrant and golden, about 2 minutes more.

2. Stir in the coconut milk, lime zest and juice, remaining salt, and pepper to taste with ½ cup water. Bring the liquid to a simmer, then cover and transfer the pot to the oven. Cook, turning the meat after an hour, until the beef is very tender, 2 to 2½ hours. Serve garnished with the cilantro and scallions, and lime wedges on the side for serving.

What Else?

- The combination of beef and coconut milk makes this dish very rich and filled with a layer of good, flavorful fat. If you'd rather skim off the fat, make

[CONTINUED]

it several hours or even a few days ahead to give the fat time to rise to the surface, then skim it off.

- Half the time I don't bother peeling the ginger if the skin looks nice and taut and not too wrinkled. When I do peel, I use the tip of a spoon.

A Dish by Another Name

- To turn this into Coconut Curry Beef, substitute madras curry powder or garam masala for the chili powder.

COCONUT RICE AND PEAS

In our house, coconut rice is like magic. Everyone loves it and everyone will eat it without fail, regardless of diet requirements, finicky moods, temper tantrums, and the like. Daniel, who is a distance runner, calls it rocket fuel when he eats a big bowl for breakfast right before a race. And Dahlia will always consent to at least a few mouthfuls, even on her most terrible day of the terrible twos. As for me, well, I just like it, and am ever glad to brew up a batch. I particularly like the way the coconut milk's creaminess softens the deep toasty flavor of brown rice, but you can also make this with white rice (see What Else?). The peas are strictly optional, but I like the bit of color they add, especially if you are serving this with the very brown coconut beef on page 46.

Serves 4

1 (13.5-ounce) can coconut milk
1 cup brown rice, rinsed
Large pinch kosher salt
3/4 cup frozen peas (optional)

1. Pour the coconut milk into a liquid measuring cup. Add enough water until the liquid measures 2 cups and pour into a large saucepan with the rice. Bring the liquid just to a boil and add the salt.
2. Reduce the heat and allow the rice to simmer until the liquid has been absorbed and the rice is tender, 45 minutes to an hour. Stir in the peas during the last 2 minutes of cooking. If the rice is tender but there is still liquid in the pan, remove the cover and simmer on high heat until the liquid evaporates. Fluff well before serving.

What Else?

- Obviously frozen peas aren't seasonal, but they add such great color, and the little morsels of sweetness are extremely welcome amidst the spicy chili sauce if you serve it with the coconut beef. However, if you'd rather not use them, just leave them out. I always leave them out when I make this for Daniel to eat for breakfast before a race. Sometimes I'll even drizzle a little maple syrup into leftovers to make an impromptu rice pudding.

- If you are making this in pea season, use fresh peas in place of frozen, and add them about 6 minutes before the rice is done.

- Or skip the peas and stir in some chopped-up (or baby) spinach leaves. Use about 2 packed cups and stir it in during the last 5 minutes of cooking as you would the peas.

- You can substitute white rice here; just reduce the cooking time to 20 minutes. You might want to cut back on the water you're adding, too. Fill the measuring cup to just shy of 2 cups—$1\frac{7}{8}$ cups works well.

- Adding a small piece of cinnamon stick, about $1\frac{1}{2}$ inches, to the pot adds a warm scent that pairs beautifully with the exotic flavors of the beef.

FRAGRANT LENTIL RICE SOUP WITH SPINACH AND CRISPY ONIONS

There are times when I want a simple, quiet lentil soup with plenty of broth and a gentle, earthy flavor. That is when I reach for my old standby, a red lentil soup with lemon recipe that I published in the *New York Times* several years ago (and you can still find it online).

But there are other, hungrier times when I want something supremely hearty and fortifying. I crave a soup that will steel me for a brisk walk on a crisp, cold February evening, the kind of meander I used to take, prebaby, whenever I felt like getting a little air after dinner and contemplating the stars. These days, my postprandial walk is more likely to be a trip to the curb with the trash. No matter—this thick, nubby soup will brace my body for any endeavor.

Made from red lentils, rice, caramelized sweet onions, and a few choice, heady spices, it's a complex, thick mix just on the soupy side of stew. A handful of spinach wilted in at the end adds color and transforms a simple soup into a handsome one-pot meal. Leftovers are even better for lunch the next day when the flavors have had a chance to marry. If there's only a little left in the pot, serve it up with a fried egg on top for a breakfast that will keep you going nearly all day long—even if you don't have to leave the house.

Serves 6

FOR THE CRISPY ONIONS

3 medium onions, halved from root to stem and thinly sliced
2 tablespoons unsalted butter
3 tablespoons olive oil
Pinch kosher salt

[CONTINUED]

2 tablespoons olive oil

1 onion, finely chopped

2-inch piece fresh gingerroot, peeled and finely chopped

2 garlic cloves, finely chopped

1 cinnamon stick

3/4 teaspoon ground cumin

Pinch ground allspice

1 bay leaf

6 cups chicken or vegetable stock

1/2 cup brown basmati rice

1 1/2 teaspoons kosher salt, more to taste

1 1/2 cups red lentils

5 ounces baby spinach leaves (about 4 cups)

1/4 cup chopped fresh mint (optional)

Lime wedges, for serving

Flaky sea salt, for serving

1. To make the onions, melt the butter and 2 tablespoons oil in a large skillet over medium-low heat. Toss in the onions. Cook 5 minutes until they begin to release their juices. Raise the heat to medium-high and continue cooking until the onions are soft and golden, about 7 minutes. Add the remaining tablespoon oil and salt and increase the heat to high. Cook, stirring only a few times, until the onions are crisp and charred in places, 5 to 10 minutes.

2. Make the soup: Heat the oil in a large pot over medium heat. Add the onion and cook, stirring, until softened, 5 to 7 minutes. Drop in the ginger, garlic, cinnamon, cumin, allspice, and bay leaf and cook until the mixture is fragrant, about 1 minute. Stir in the stock, 3 cups water, the rice, and the salt. Bring to a boil over high heat, then immediately reduce the flame to medium-low and let the rice simmer for 10 minutes. Stir in the red lentils and cook until the rice is tender and the lentils are meltingly soft, about 30 minutes. Stir in the spinach and 2 tablespoons mint if using and let them wilt completely.

Taste and add more salt if necessary. If the dish tastes flat, squeeze in a lime wedge or two.

3. Ladle the soup into serving bowls and top with a small handful of crispy onions. Garnish with the remaining mint if desired and a sprinkling of flaky salt. Serve with lime wedges.

What Else?

- If you don't eat up this soup in one go, you can stir in all the onions before refrigerating the soup.

- If you like your soup on the brothy side, just add a little more water or stock at the end of cooking.

- Buttery paratha (page 278) makes an excellent accompaniment, and you can whip up the flatbread while the soup simmers.

- Swiss chard or kale can be substituted for the spinach, though they might need to simmer for a few extra minutes to soften.

SLICED ORANGES WITH OLIVES AND RED CHILE

Somewhere along the way in my life, I learned how to supreme an orange. This technique lets me run my knife under the fruit's skin to remove it all, along with the bitter pith, in one fell swoop. It made orange peeling instant, easy, and—in the rare moment when I actually had one—not manicure massacring. Plus, this new trick gave me license to add oranges to everything that screamed out for a bit of brightness and sweet juice. Even just serving the sunny-colored slices laid out on a plate, drizzled with good olive oil and sprinkled with salt, elevated the typical orange snack to a salad of utter delight.

I serve this on days when I can't be bothered to wash salad greens or when there aren't any in the fridge. It's also marvelous dinner party fare since it's refreshing after a large meal, easy to make ahead, can sit out on a buffet for hours if necessary, and is completely and utterly unexpected. If you are going to make this for a party, use a combination of citrus for the prettiest salad imaginable.

3 large oranges, preferably a combination of orange navel, pink Cara Cara, and blood orange (see What Else?)
Good extra-virgin olive oil
Flaky sea salt
3 tablespoons thinly sliced olives (use your favorite kind)
Some kind of chili powder to taste
Chopped fresh herbs, if you want the added color

Serves 4

1. Trim off the top and bottom of an orange so it can stand upright on the cutting board. Use a thin, sharp knife to slice off the peel and white pith, following the curve of the fruit as you go. The juicy orange flesh should be exposed. Turn the orange so the curved side is lying on the board, then thinly slice the orange 1/4 inch thick. The slices should look a little like flowers. Repeat with the remaining oranges.

2. Spread the orange slices on a large plate, overlapping them somewhat but not entirely. Drizzle with plenty of the good oil and sprinkle with sea salt. Top with the olives and dust with chili right before serving. Sprinkle with chopped herbs, if you like.

What Else?

- This salad really is sunset pretty if you use all three kinds of oranges. But use whatever you can get.

- If you're serving more people, just slice up a few more oranges. You can also try throwing pink and white grapefruits, tangerines, and pomelos into the mix to give the widest possible variety of color.

- Chopped olives, sliced scallions or sweet onions, toasted almonds, ground cinnamon or nutmeg, orange blossom water, sliced dates, parsley leaves, minced garlic, and chopped anchovies are some other options that can go on top of the oranges. Mix and match, using your discretion.

CREAMY PARSNIP AND LEEK SOUP WITH PUMPERNICKEL CROUTONS

Bone-chilling, damp days and frosty nights bellow for soup, so in February we eat pots upon pots of it. And one of my favorite midweek, postwork, didn't-plan-anything-else-for-dinner soups to throw together is a simple root vegetable puree.

My technique never varies, and it always produces something good and heartwarming to eat.

I start with a sautéed base of alliums (onion, shallot, leek, garlic, whatever-have-you), add whatever root vegetables are starting to soften in the bin, some kind of seasonings (herbs, spices), and plenty of good, preferably homemade broth (or water seasoned with a lot of salt and pepper). Then I let everything simmer until the roots are spoonably soft. The final puree is as creamy and comforting as mashed potatoes, but eminently more meal-like and satisfying.

The parsnips and leeks in this version make it sweeter and milder than most, so I like to pair it with something bright flavored and bold. Crusty dark bread, toasted and rubbed with garlic, is a simple, crunchy, bold contrast to the pale suppleness of the soup. A simple salad of whatever greens you've got will round out your meal.

Serves 4 to 6

4 to 6 tablespoons butter
4 large leeks, white and light green parts only, cleaned and sliced
    (see What Else?)
1 teaspoon kosher salt, more to taste
Plenty of freshly ground black pepper
4 large celery stalks with leaves
4 thyme sprigs
1 bay leaf
Parsley stems, if you've got them (optional)

1¼ pounds parsnips, peeled and sliced

1 pound potatoes (2 to 3 small ones), peeled and chunked

1 quart chicken or vegetable broth

Few drops fresh lemon juice, if needed

Thick slices pumpernickel or other hearty bread

1 garlic clove, halved

Good olive oil, for drizzling

Turkish or Syrian red pepper, such as Aleppo, for dusting (see What Else?)

1. Melt the butter in a soup pot, then add the leeks, salt, and black pepper and sauté gently over medium heat until the leeks are softened, about 5 minutes.

2. Meanwhile, slice the celery, reserving the leaves. Add the celery to the pot and continue to sauté for another 5 minutes, until the leeks are lightly golden around the edges and the celery is shiny.

3. If you've got kitchen twine, tie the thyme, bay leaf, and celery leaves into a bundle (you could also add parsley stems here if you like). Throw it into the pot along with the parsnips, potatoes, and broth (if you don't have twine, just throw in the herbs, but you will have to fish them out later). Add 2 cups of water and bring everything to a simmer; let cook until the vegetables are perfectly soft without any hard bits, 30 to 45 minutes.

4. Pluck out and discard the herbs or herb bundle. Puree the soup, adding a little water if it seems too thick. Add more salt to taste and some lemon juice if the flavor seems a little flat.

5. To serve, toast the bread, then rub with the garlic halves and drizzle with oil. Ladle the soup into bowls and garnish with olive oil and red pepper.

What Else?

- To clean leeks, slice them in half lengthwise. Holding each leek half under a running tap, let the water slide between the leek layers, swishing out any soil hidden there.

[CONTINUED]

- Yes, you can skip the red pepper or substitute chili powder. I wouldn't, but then again I am so addicted to my sticky, spicy, fruity Turkish red pepper that I keep a miniature porcelain tagine full of it on my dining table, and add it to any food that needs a little *something*. You might call this my secret weapon, which I brandish whenever I can't think of what else to add to take a dish from good to amazing. One sprinkle, usually in tandem with some flaky sea salt and a drizzle of excellent olive oil, usually does the trick. I got into the habit of red pepper sprinkling when Daniel and I visited Turkey. It was as ubiquitous as black pepper is in American cooking, and it deepened the flavor of everything from yogurt to kebabs to the most ornate of pilafs. Aleppo pepper, from nearby Syria, is another favorite, with a slightly smokier flavor. You can order both from any spice store.

A Dish by Another Name

- For Creamy Celery Root and Leek Soup: Substitute 2 pounds celery root for the parsnips. To make Double Celery Soup, omit the potato and bump up the celery stalks quotient to 5 or 6. Garnish with chopped celery leaves.

- For Creamy Parsnip and Leek Soup with Crispy Bacon: Omit the butter. In the soup pot, fry diced bacon until crisp, then drain on paper towels. Sauté the vegetables in the bacon fat and proceed with the recipe as directed, garnishing with the bacon bits just before serving so they stay crisp.

BUTTERY, GARLICKY, SPICY CALAMARI WITH ISRAELI COUSCOUS

When most people think of cheap, fast food, they think of drive-through burgers. When I think of fast food, I think of calamari. It's probably one of the least expensive, tastiest, quickest-cooking sea creatures out there, all the while being sustainable and plentiful, so there's no reason not to eat it all the time. Which we do.

The squid I buy at the fish store is a snap to cook with because it comes well cleaned. I slice up the bodies while the oil heats, and this dish is ready in under 10 minutes.

The squid from the farmers' market, however, demands a bit more attention since it comes straight off the fishing boat and can be sandy. I give it a strong rinse under lots of cold water to dislodge lingering grit (make sure to flush out the cavity). The clean, ocean flavor of this uber-fresh squid makes it worth the extra sand-removal effort.

Once you've got your squid in order, this dish really does cook in minutes, so make sure you have everything else on the table—the salad in the bowl waiting to be tossed with vinaigrette, the wine poured, and the candles lit (yes, this dish is candleworthy)—before you starting heating the pan. In minutes, you'll serve a savory, garlicky, herb-flecked squid to your favorite people, who couldn't be happier had you slaved at the stove all day long.

Serves 4

1¹/₂ cups Israeli couscous

2¹/₂ tablespoons olive oil

1¹/₂ pounds squid, cut into ¹/₂-inch pieces and patted as dry as you can get it

3 tablespoons unsalted butter

2 tablespoons chopped fresh parsley

1 tablespoon chopped fresh basil

[CONTINUED]

Large pinch (or 2) red pepper flakes

3 large garlic cloves, minced

Large pinch coarse kosher salt

Large pinch freshly ground black pepper

Freshly squeezed lemon juice to taste

1. In a large pot of boiling salted water, cook the couscous until tender, 4 to 5 minutes. Drain well, toss with $1/2$ tablespoon olive oil, and keep warm.

2. In a very large skillet over high heat, heat the remaining oil until it begins to smoke. Carefully add the squid, butter, parsley, basil, red pepper flakes, and garlic (if your pan is small you may have to do this in two batches; you don't want it too full to toss). Cook, tossing frequently, until the squid is opaque and cooked through, 3 to 4 minutes. Season to taste with salt, pepper, and lemon juice. Add the couscous to the pan and toss until incorporated.

What Else?

- We love this dish so much we've eaten it almost every which way—over pasta, rice, regular couscous, polenta, with toasted country bread, with roasted potatoes, you name it. Large pearls of Israeli couscous are our favorite; there is something thrilling about the way the slippery orbs surround the pieces of squid in your mouth like little bubbles, making the whole thing seem effervescent on the tongue. Fregola, which is similar to Israeli couscous but toasted, is a fine substitute if you see it. If you can't get either one, linguine, either whole wheat or regular semolina, is our second choice, with toasted country bread a close third. Really, you could serve a mound of feathers with this and it would still taste amazing. It's just really, really good.

- Feel free to vary the herbs; just stick to soft, floppy herbs such as mint, lovage, celery leaves, chervil, chives, and cilantro. If you do want to use branchy herbs such as rosemary, oregano, or thyme, you will have to de-stem and chop them finely before adding to the pan. The cooking time is too quick to allow anything on a stem to lend enough flavor to the oil.

- You can cook shrimp using this same technique, and it is terrific. Choose small shrimp, or slice large ones in half so they cook quickly and evenly.

- Ditto scallops. Cut large sea scallops in half, or use small bay scallops; just be sure to pat them as dry as you can.

LEMONY OLIVE OIL BANANA BREAD WITH CHOCOLATE CHIPS

If you don't have bananas so speckled with brown you can barely see the yellow beneath, don't make this recipe. Hold off until you can smell the bananas in the fruit bowl from the moment you crack open the front door. When the whole house takes on that particular sweet, caramelized, vaguely decayed scent, you're ready to go.

Waiting for the bananas to turn ultra ripe before eating them all is about the hardest thing you'll need to do for this quick bread, especially if you are like me and love bananas. The recipe itself couldn't be more straightforward. The whole wheat adds a slightly warm, toasty flavor that works nicely with the sugary bananas. And the olive oil gives it a toehold on the savory side, while still calling the sweet side home.

It's the kind of thing you can throw together on a lazy Sunday afternoon while playing with the baby at the same time (sit her at your feet, give her measuring spoons and banana peels to play with, ignore the mess). You'll be glad to eat your cake for teatime snacks all week long.

Serves 8 to 10

1 cup all-purpose flour

1 cup whole wheat flour

3/4 cup dark brown sugar

3/4 teaspoon baking soda

1/2 teaspoon kosher salt

1 cup coarsely chopped bittersweet chocolate

1/3 cup extra-virgin olive oil

2 large eggs, lightly beaten

1 1/2 cups mashed, VERY ripe bananas (3 to 4 bananas)

1/4 cup sour cream or plain whole milk yogurt

1 teaspoon freshly grated lemon zest
1 teaspoon vanilla extract

FOR THE GLAZE
1 cup confectioners' sugar
4 teaspoons freshly squeezed lemon juice

1. Preheat the oven to 350°F. Grease a 9×5-inch loaf pan.
2. In a large bowl, whisk together the flours, brown sugar, baking soda, and salt. Add the chocolate pieces and combine well.
3. In a separate bowl, mix together the olive oil, eggs, mashed bananas, sour cream or yogurt, lemon zest, and vanilla. Pour the banana mixture into the flour mixture and fold with a spatula until just combined. Scrape the batter into the prepared pan and bake until dark golden brown and a tester inserted into the middle of the loaf comes out clean, 50 minutes to 1 hour.
4. Transfer the pan to a wire rack over a rimmed baking sheet to cool in the pan for 10 minutes, then turn the loaf out of the pan to cool completely.
5. While the cake is almost cool, prepare the glaze. In a bowl, whisk together the confectioners' sugar and lemon juice until smooth. Drizzle the glaze on top of the cake, spreading with a spatula to cover.

What Else?

- Like most banana breads and nearly all sweet muffins, this is really cake in disguise. I'm calling it by its traditional designation so you'll know exactly what I'm talking about. But don't let the recipe title fool you. Serve this for dessert or a sweet afternoon nibble.

- If you don't like lemons or don't like glazes, skip the glaze. Without it, the bread will be less cakelike and more classically banana bread-ish.

[CONTINUED]

- Ditto for the chocolate chips. Walnuts make a traditional and nice substitute for them.

- If you want it even sweeter and more cakelike, substitute melted butter for the olive oil. Safflower and canola oil also work for a more neutral-tasting cake.

TINY VALENTINE'S DAY CAKE FOR DANIEL (DEVIL'S FOOD CAKE WITH BUTTER RUM FROSTING)

I acquired my first 6-inch cake pan when I made the wedding cake for two friends in graduate school. It was a casual affair, a quick jaunt to City Hall followed by a reception at someone's apartment. My job was to make a tiered chocolate cake with white buttercream, covered in flowers.

At this point in my baking career I'd never quadrupled a cake recipe, never cut dowels to stack cake layers on top of each other, and had never tried to frost anything more ambitious than a birthday cake.

But I bumbled my way through it, obsessively reading and rereading the assembly instructions in Rose Levy Beranbaum's book *The Cake Bible*, making sure to have a lot of extra icing and big bright flowers on hand to disguise potential disasters.

Well, let's just say that first cake was a good lesson in why professionally made cakes cost what they do. Even my ugly-duck cake was scarily time consuming, especially because I'd forgotten to mix the baking powder into the first batch of batter I put in the oven. Then, for all my efforts, the poor cake was lopsided and hunchbacked, its pristine white icing strewn here and there with nubby black crumbs I couldn't mask, and covered, willy-nilly, with slightly wilted gerbera daisies. The maid of honor said it was rustic and homemade looking, and I know she meant it as a compliment. Luckily, it hardly mattered. The bride and groom stopped at a bar on the way to the reception, and drank so many congratulatory shots that when they finally showed up, they barely noticed the cake, which all the tipsy guests devoured with their hands when we ran out of forks.

Since then, my friends have divorced and remarried, and I have drastically improved my cake-making skills (and plastic fork–buying skills). I've made four

[CONTINUED]

more wedding cakes (never my own, by the way), and all were lovely and not at all lopsided, if still pleasingly homemade looking and rustic.

All this is to say that those 6-inch cake pans I bought for a wedding cake back in my student days have been put to good use, and not just for wedding cakes. I also love using them to bake tiny layer cakes to feed four to six people. Or in this Valentine's Day recipe, two, with ample leftovers for breakfast the next morning.

FOR THE CHOCOLATE CAKE

Serves 4 to 6
(or 2 with leftovers)

2/3 cup very hot coffee or water

1/3 cup unsweetened, Dutch process cocoa powder

3/4 teaspoon kosher salt

4 large egg yolks (save the whites for the buttercream)

1 tablespoon vanilla extract

1 1/2 cups cake flour

2 teaspoons baking powder

1 stick (8 tablespoons) unsalted butter, softened

1 cup sugar

1 cup chopped sweet and spicy candied pecans (page 365)
    or purchased toffee bits (optional)

FOR THE RUM BUTTERCREAM

4 large egg whites

1 cup sugar

1/4 teaspoon kosher salt

3 sticks unsalted butter (12 ounces), at room temperature, sliced

3 tablespoons good aged rum

1. Preheat the oven to 350°F. Grease and flour two 6-inch pans, or spray with baking spray. Cut parchment or wax paper rounds to fit in the bottom of the pans, lay them down, and grease the paper.

2. In a small bowl, stir together the coffee and cocoa until smooth. Stir in the salt and let cool until barely warm to the touch. Whisk in the egg yolks and vanilla.

3. In a large bowl, whisk together the flour and baking powder.

4. Using an electric mixer, beat the butter until fluffy. Add the sugar and continue to beat until very light, about 5 minutes. Beat in a third of the cocoa mixture, followed by half of the flour mixture, and beat well. Scrape down the sides of the mixer and beat again. Beat in another third of the cocoa mixture and then the remaining flour mixture. Scrape the sides again and add the remaining cocoa. Beat until smooth.

5. Divide the batter evenly between the two cake pans and smooth the tops. Bake until the tops of the cakes are no longer shiny and wet looking, and a cake tester inserted in the center emerges clean, 30 to 35 minutes. Cool on wire racks before unmolding.

6. To prepare the buttercream, put the egg whites, sugar, and salt into the metal bowl of your mixer (or any metal bowl if using a handheld mixer). Bring a medium pot of water to a boil. Place the bowl of egg whites over the pot and whisk until the sugar is dissolved and the eggs are warm to the touch. Use pot holders if necessary to hold on to the bowl.

7. Remove the bowl from the heat and beat the eggs with an electric mixer until they are thick and cool, about 5 minutes (see What Else? for tips). Beat in the butter, bit by bit, until the mixture is smooth and fluffy and buttercreamy. Beat in the rum. Use immediately, or store at room temperature for up to 24 hours. You might have to beat it again before using.

8. If the cakes are quite domed on top, use a knife to slice off the humps so the cake will be level (this is what professionals do to get perfectly even layers). Slice the cakes in half horizontally, and spread the buttercream between the layers, adding some of the chopped nuts or toffee bits if you like. Ice the cake, then cover with more of the nuts or toffee.

What Else?

- If you don't want to use toffee bits or candied nuts in the cake, you can use plain toasted nuts instead (any kind you like; hazelnuts are nice with rum). Or leave out the crunch altogether, as this recipe really doesn't need it.

[CONTINUED]

- Or if you'd rather, bake the batter in a 9-inch pan. The baking time may differ, so start checking it after 25 minutes.

- One thing I learned from that first wedding-cake experience was to lock the crumbs onto the cake by sealing it with a thin layer of icing before adding the rest. To do this, put about a third of your icing into a separate bowl and use it to apply a thin layer of frosting. When all the crumbs are locked into that first layer of icing, clean your spatula and apply a second layer of frosting on top. If you have the time and fridge space to chill your cake layers in between applying the first and second coats of icing, definitely do so. It will make everything neater and easier.

- Large, colorful flowers still work as a distracting, pretty decoration for the cake, especially on Valentine's Day.

- The biggest thing to pay attention to when making a meringue buttercream—technically what this recipe is—is the temperature of the ingredients. The butter really needs to be soft, pliable, and at room temperature, not melty, not hard, and not cold. So make sure to take it out of the fridge an hour before you plan to make this. If you've only got half an hour, you can cheat by slicing the butter into slices and spreading those out on a plate. They will warm faster this way. Don't use the microwave unless you are very careful, because chances are the butter will melt.

  Then there is the temperature of the egg whites. They must be completely cool, not warm, when you add the butter. Basically, in order to form the most stable emulsion, you want the butter and egg whites to be the same temperature. If one is too cold, the mixture will curdle. If one is too hot, the mixture will melt into soup. If, in spite of your best effots, you end up with liquidy, thin buttercream, set it briefly in a bowl of ice water, then try beating it again. If everything gets curdled, set the bowl in a bowl of very warm (not hot) water and try beating it again. You can usually rescue broken buttercream, but it will take some doing.

MARCH

GINGERY SPLIT PEA SOUP
WITH TOASTED CORIANDER

*"Pease porridge hot, pease porridge cold,
 pease porridge in the pot, nine days old . . ."*

Maybe it's the nursery rhyme that put it in my head that pea soup is necessarily porridge thick, but because of that, I've largely avoided split pea soup.

It's not that I don't like porridge. I eat hot cereal for breakfast on most winter mornings. And it's not that I don't like split peas. A spiced dal, perfumed with ginger and coriander and runny enough to soak into a basmati rice pilaf, is one of my favorite aspects of an Indian meal.

When I realized I could bring some of the spices I love in dal to a split pea soup, I knew I just might have a pea soup that I could dream about and heartily enjoy.

Still, one thing I discovered when I finally tried to make my own split pea soup is that no matter how much water and stock you add to the peas, as soon they cool, they thicken into a solid mass. But fixing it is easy; just add stock or water while stirring it over a low flame until it turns back into a liquid.

Or, even better, eat it all up while it's still hot. And with this zesty soup, flavored with aromatic herbs, spicy ginger, and a brightening, sunshiny jolt of lemon zest and juice, finishing the pot shouldn't be any problem.

1 teaspoon whole coriander seed, crushed with the flat side of a knife
    (or use 1 teaspoon ground coriander)
1 1/2 tablespoons olive oil
2 carrots, peeled and chopped
1 celery stalk with leaves, chopped
1 large onion, chopped
1 medium leek, white and light green parts only, chopped
4 garlic cloves, chopped

Serves 4

2-inch-thick piece of gingerroot, peeled and grated

1 pound split peas, picked over and rinsed

6 cups chicken or vegetable stock

2 teaspoons kosher salt, more to taste

1/4 teaspoon freshly ground black pepper

2 rosemary branches, plus additional chopped leaves,
    for garnish

1 bay leaf

1/2 teaspoon finely grated lemon zest

Freshly squeezed juice of 1/2 lemon

Good olive oil, for drizzling

1. In a large saucepan over medium-high heat, toast the coriander until fragrant, 1 to 2 minutes, then pour in the oil. Stir in the carrots, celery, onion, leek, garlic, and ginger. Reduce the heat to medium; cook, stirring, until the vegetables are softened, about 5 minutes.

2. Stir in the peas, 4 cups water, the stock, salt, and pepper. Drop in the rosemary and bay leaf (you can tie them up in kitchen string if you like; this makes them easier to remove later). Bring the soup to a boil over medium-high heat. Reduce the heat to medium-low; simmer until the peas are tender and falling apart and the soup is thick, about 1 1/2 hours. Remove and discard the rosemary and bay leaf. Stir in the lemon zest and juice.

3. Thin with water to the desired consistency. Warm over medium-low heat if need be. Ladle into bowls; drizzle with oil and garnish with chopped rosemary.

What Else?

- You can use either all leeks or all onions if it's easier. I used one of each because that's what I had around.

- If you are a lover of thick, porridge-like pea soups, use a little less water. Then serve the dish over rice as a pea stew, with some sautéed greens on

[CONTINUED]

the side for a full meal. Browned onions (page 51) would make a fine garnish for a pea stew.

• If you absolutely hate split peas, try making this with red lentils instead. It
will be brothier and lighter than the pea version, but just as savory.

BUTTER LETTUCE AND CLEMENTINE SALAD WITH BROWN BUTTER VINAIGRETTE

I'm very suggestible when it comes to food, which is probably why, for years, I've had the itch to dress a butter lettuce salad with a butter-based vinaigrette.

But I'd never seen a recipe for a butter-based vinaigrette, so I assumed some earlier culinary pioneer had been there, done that, and decided, after all, that it wasn't a very good idea.

Then I wrote an article on chefs cooking with brown butter for the *New York Times.* And I learned that besides using it in rich pan sauces for fish and brains, some chefs made brown butter into vinaigrette to dress seafood and hearty salads.

The trick to keeping the butter from solidifying is to add just enough very potent liquid—either citrus juice or vinegar—to add flavor and keep everything flowing without diluting the nutty flavor of the browned butter. I used clementine juice because I always keep clementines in the fridge in winter (Dahlia and I both love how easy they are to pull apart and stuff into one's mouth), but oranges or other tangerines would work as well.

And you know what? Brown butter vinaigrette on butter lettuce is quite wonderful, especially when it's also tossed with toasted almonds, fresh mint, and bright clementine segments. Even Dahlia will eat this, which is saying a lot when it comes to two-year-olds and salad.

Serves 2 to 4

FOR THE VINAIGRETTE

3 tablespoons unsalted butter

Finely grated zest of 1 clementine

1½ tablespoons freshly squeezed clementine juice

1 tablespoon freshly squeezed lemon juice

[CONTINUED]

¼ teaspoon kosher salt

Freshly ground black pepper to taste

FOR THE BUTTER LETTUCE SALAD

1 head butter leaf lettuce, leaves torn into bite-size pieces

2 clementines, peeled, segmented, segments cut in half crosswise

2 tablespoons toasted almonds

2 tablespoons chopped fresh mint

1. Make the vinaigrette: In a small skillet over medium-low heat, melt the butter. Cook the butter gently until it turns nut brown, about 5 minutes. Watch it carefully to see that it does not burn. Immediately pour into a bowl and let cool to room temperature (if it's a cold room and it solidifies, just pop it in the microwave for a few seconds). Whisk in the clementine zest and juice, the lemon juice, salt, and pepper.

2. In a large bowl, combine the lettuce, clementine segments, almonds, and mint. Drizzle the vinaigrette over the salad and toss well.

What Else?

- The combination of clementines, almonds, and butter lettuce is so good, it's worth making even if you're not in the mood to make a brown butter vinaigrette (which isn't hard to do, but requires an extra step compared to an olive oil vinaigrette). So go ahead and substitute olive oil for the butter (no need to heat it). Or, to mimic the nutty flavor that the toasted butter imparts, you could mix half olive oil with half hazelnut oil.

- This is a rare occurrence where I prefer my citrus broken up into segments instead of being supremed and stripped down to their juicy parts (see page 54). And that's because the small pieces of clementine sections keep their juice to themselves—until you bite in and get a juicy burst of sweet-tart flavor on the tongue. Since a large part of the clementine's appeal here is its daintiness, if you do need to substitute another citrus fruit, cut the segments into thirds or fourths, then add them to the lettuce after it's already been tossed with vinaigrette. Gently toss again and serve immediately. This will preserve as much of the juice in the sections as possible, without it leaking all over the lettuce and diluting the richness of the brown butter dressing.

BRAISED PORK SHOULDER WITH TOMATOES, CINNAMON, AND OLIVES OVER POLENTA

This is exactly the right kind of savory, warming dish to bring to a friend who is feeling unwell. Or at least, that's why I made it last winter.

It was for Josh, who was just back home from the hospital after being hit by a car while riding his bike. His wrist was smashed to bits, and he would need a year of surgeries before he fully recovered. But more important, his spirit was shaken. He vacillated between feelings of terror (he really could have died), anger (why was that *&$%&* car service driver speeding up Eighth Avenue anyway?), intense gratitude (for being alive), and deep love for his family (his wife, Bryony, and toddler daughter, Willa).

Josh needed many things and nothing from his friends in those fragile, postaccident days, including excellent, soul-sustaining meals. That was right up my alley.

Naturally, I wanted to make him something special, but didn't know what.

So I wandered the farmers' market stalls that morning, looking for inspiration, which unveiled itself to me in the form of a small chunk of pork shoulder. Offering various shoulders to Josh and family—to cry on, to eat—seemed apropos for this particular situation, so I snapped it right up.

With a pork shoulder in the bag, a cook has options. I could have roasted it surrounded by the season's last root vegetables. But by this point in the season, I was tiring of root vegetables. And a braise is always easier to transport and reheat than a roast.

For the seasonings, I wanted to simmer up something comforting but different, something vaguely exotic that would taste of sunny, faraway places where no one ever drove SUVs at top speed down residential streets.

I doubt this place exists, but if it does, I'm sure they use plenty of dry red wine and sweet spices in their braises, along with anchovies for complexity, and tart olives and those canned plum tomatoes I had in the cupboard as a bright contrast.

I cooked it carefully and brought it over to Josh's house with some freshly made polenta and a chilled bottle of Champagne. Because this dinner was a celebration—of luck, pork, dedicated bike lanes, and most important, eating good food with dear friends.

Serves 4 to 6

2 pounds pork shoulder (also called pork butt),
    cut into 2-inch chunks
Kosher salt and freshly ground black pepper, for seasoning
2 tablespoons olive oil
2 large leeks, white and light green parts only, sliced
5 garlic cloves, smashed and peeled
1 (28-ounce) can plum tomatoes
1 cup dry red wine
5 anchovies
2-inch piece cinnamon stick
2 bay leaves
2 rosemary sprigs
$2/3$ cup pitted and roughly chopped green olives
Cooked polenta, for serving (see What Else? page 270)

1. Preheat the oven to 300°F. Season the pork shoulder generously with salt and pepper. In a Dutch oven over medium-high heat, warm the olive oil and sear the pork, turning, until it is well browned all over, about 10 minutes. Transfer the pork to a plate.

2. Add the leeks and garlic to the Dutch oven and brown, stirring, 3 to 5 minutes.

3. Return the pork to the Dutch oven and add the tomatoes, wine, anchovies, cinnamon stick, bay leaves, and rosemary. Cover the Dutch oven and place it in the oven. Cook for 1½ to 2 hours, turning the pork twice during cooking (once after 45 minutes and again after an hour and a half).

[CONTINUED]

4. Raise the temperature to 425°F. Uncover the Dutch oven and add the olives. Continue cooking, uncovered, until the liquid is reduced and the meat is very tender, about 20 minutes more. If you have made this ahead of time, let it cool so the fat has a chance to rise to the surface, then spoon it off if you like (I usually don't bother). If you've made it the day before, chilling hardens the fat and makes it really easy to spoon off. Reheat if necessary and serve over polenta.

What Else?

- I don't know why pork shoulder is also called the butt, or sometimes Boston butt. All I do know is that it's an ideal cut for braising because the meat is shot through with gelatin and fat, which melts when cooked at low heat, moistening and tenderizing the pork. It's also extremely inexpensive, at least compared to other, fancier cuts like tenderloin.

- The flavors and cooking technique in this dish work beautifully with lamb. Substitute boneless lamb shoulder for the pork and proceed with the recipe as written.

- Like nearly all braised foods, this dish reheats nicely, so feel free to make it a couple of days ahead and refrigerate. Reheat it on the stove over very low heat until the sauce bubbles and the meat is warmed through.

- Warm, nubby barley is another terrific accompaniment to this dish. Try the recipe on page 125, or follow the directions on the package.

MUSTARD GREENS SALAD WITH ANCHOVY CROUTONS AND GRUYÈRE CHEESE

Small, purple-tinged leaves of baby mustard greens are wonderful in salads, where they add both a spicy note and a vivid, contrasting color. I first noticed them in a salad mix that one of the farmers at the market sold, and once I tried them I was hooked.

I bought the mix for years before it occurred to me to try just buying the mini mustard greens and making a salad out of those alone. I knew it would be pungent, so I tossed in lots of grated cheese and croutons to add richness and cut the heat. I also threw in anchovies because their salty assertiveness tends to go well with other strong flavors. And I adore anchovies in salads—Caesar and otherwise.

Because of its richness, this isn't the best salad to offer after a heavy entrée in the French salad-after-main-course mode. But don't let that stop you from whipping it up to serve as an appetizer. It's also hearty enough to munch on its own for lunch, which is how I usually eat it.

Serves 4 as an appetizer or 2 for lunch

2 fat garlic cloves, finely chopped

1/8 teaspoon plus 1 pinch kosher salt, more to taste

1/3 cup extra-virgin olive oil

4 anchovy fillets, finely chopped

1/4 teaspoon freshly ground black pepper

5 ounces crusty bread, cut into 3/4-inch cubes (about 3 cups)

1/4 pound Gruyère cheese, grated (about 1 cup), optional

5 ounces mustard greens, preferably baby greens (about 6 cups loosely packed)

4 teaspoons freshly squeezed lemon juice

[CONTINUED]

1. Preheat the oven to 375°F.
2. With a mortar and pestle or using the side of a knife, mash the garlic with a pinch of salt. Transfer to a small bowl. Whisk in the oil, anchovies, 1/8 teaspoon salt, and pepper.
3. Spread the bread cubes onto a large baking sheet. Drizzle with 2 tablespoons of the anchovy mixture and toss well. Scatter half of the cheese over the bread. Bake, tossing occasionally, until the croutons are golden and crisp, about 20 minutes.
4. While the croutons bake, remove the center ribs from the mustard greens if they are tough (nibble one to see). Slice the mustard greens into 1/2-inch strips. Transfer to a large bowl.
5. Whisk the lemon juice into the remaining anchovy oil. Pour the remaining vinaigrette over the greens and toss to combine. Add the croutons and remaining cheese to the salad; toss gently. Taste and adjust the seasonings, if necessary.

What Else?

- If you can't get baby—or at least teenage—mustard greens for this salad, don't substitute the full-grown leaves, which are usually too bitter to eat raw. Instead use a bitter greens or Asian greens salad mix, or substitute arugula, which has a similar peppery bite to the mustard.

- Without the cheese to soften this salad, it's leaner and more intense tasting, but no less delicious. So feel free to feed it to the dairy-free.

SPICY BLACK BEANS WITH CHORIZO AND JALAPEÑOS

My college friend Mara turned me on to this dish, which she made in her dorm room on a weekly basis. Her version was minimalist. She'd warm up a can of Goya black beans, stirring a little ground cumin and oregano into the pot. Then she'd pour it over cooked rice and top it with fried eggs and hot sauce. It was satisfying, cheap, and easy enough to make while simultaneously trying to memorize the minutia of the biliary tract.

My recipe is slightly more involved. I add sautéed vegetables because I love the gentle crunch of peppers and onions amid all that carbohydrate goodness of beans and rice. The optional chorizo adds spice and meatiness to what is otherwise one of the heartier of vegetarian entrées. Best of all, it's still satisfying, cheap, and easy enough to make while wrangling a toddler underfoot—which may or may not be easier than collegiate biology.

Serves 2

2 tablespoons extra-virgin olive oil

3 ounces cured chorizo, cut into $1/2$-inch cubes (optional)

1 Vidalia or other sweet onion, diced

2 large garlic cloves, finely chopped

1 red bell pepper, diced

1 jalapeño, seeded and finely chopped

$3/4$ teaspoon dried oregano

$3/4$ teaspoon ground cumin

1 (15.5-ounce) can black beans, drained but not rinsed

$3/4$ teaspoon kosher salt

3 tablespoons chopped fresh cilantro

Hot sauce to taste

Cooked brown or white rice, for serving

2 fried eggs, for serving (optional)

[CONTINUED]

1. In a large skillet over medium-high heat, warm the oil. Add the chorizo and cook until light golden, about 3 minutes. Stir in the onion, garlic, pepper, and jalapeño. Cook, stirring, until the vegetables are softened, about 7 minutes. Stir in the oregano and cumin; cook 1 minute more. Stir in the beans and salt and simmer gently for 5 minutes.
2. Remove the pot from the heat. Stir in the cilantro and hot sauce. Serve over rice. Top each plate with a fried egg, if desired.

What Else?

- Cured chorizo is a salted and dried version of the famous Spanish sausage, with a similar texture to salami. You can substitute fresh (raw) chorizo, but you will only need to use 1 tablespoon of oil to sauté it. Remove the casings and then break apart the chorizo meat as you sauté it, making sure it cooks through and browns all over. Fresh hot Italian sausage is also an option here if that's all you can find. Or, if you'd rather retain the chewy texture of the cured chorizo but can't find it, use salami or hot sopressata instead.

- Of course, you can substitute freshly cooked black beans for the canned stuff. Use about 1 3/4 cups.

WILTED COLLARD GREENS WITH LEMON AND EXTRA-VIRGIN OLIVE OIL

This is collard greens in their most pure and delicate manifestation, without ham hocks or hot sauce or chile or garlic to distract you from their sweet, grassy flavor. The greens are blanched in salted water, drained, and dressed simply, with olive oil, lemon juice, and salt—just enough to bring out their fresh taste without covering it up under the assumption that in fact you don't really like collard greens at all and you are just eating them for the meat and condiments they are cooked with.

If you meet this closet collard-hating criteria, this recipe isn't for you.

But if you love the taste of all things green, this will become a standard in your repertoire as it has for me. I especially like to make it to accompany a highly seasoned stew or pasta dish; the mellowness acts as a great foil for spicy, intense flavors. However, if you eat the collards alone and find them on the bland side, no one is going to stop you from brandishing the hot sauce bottle. The good thing about having your own kitchen, Julia Child supposedly said after she dropped a chicken on the floor, is that nobody can see what you are doing. Hail to that.

Serves 2 to 4

Kosher salt

1 large bunch collard greens, stems removed, leaves torn into pieces

2 tablespoons good olive oil, more to taste

1 tablespoon fresh lemon juice, more to taste

1. Bring a large pot of salted water to a boil. Add the collard greens and let wilt. Cook until the leaves are soft enough to please you, 2 to 7 minutes depending on the age of the greens and your desire for tenderness.

[CONTINUED]

2. Drain the collards and press out as much water as you can with a large spoon or a spatula. Put the greens in a bowl and toss with the oil, lemon juice, and salt. Adjust the seasonings to taste.

What Else?

- A few splashes of hot sauce really perk this up if you feel like something hot.

- This basic recipe will work with any kind of hearty braising green—kale, mustard, Swiss chard, broccoli rabe, even spinach, though honestly I'd probably rather eat my spinach sautéed with garlic and hot pepper flakes. But that's me.

A Dish by Another Name

- For Wilted Collard Green Salad with Feta and Olives, just add some crumbled feta and pitted black olives to the bowl. Kalamatas work particularly well here.

BAKED STUFFED POTATOES WITH CORNED BEEF AND DILL BUTTER

The only corned beef I knew from my childhood was in Jewish-style deli sandwiches, stuffed so full of meat that even after splitting mine with my sister, we still had leftovers to take home for lunch the next day. When I finally tucked into a plate of Irish corned beef and cabbage at someone's house one St. Patrick's Day in high school, it was as exotic to me as reindeer meat.

Truth be told, as much as I appreciated the soft, melting texture of the meat, potatoes, and cabbage, I can't say I ever really craved it. The whole thing was a little bland and, well, it just seemed to want a jolt of deli mustard and some rye bread to bring it all together.

Even so, every year around St. Paddy's Day, I contemplate making corned beef and cabbage just to see if maybe my opinion's changed as I've gotten older and hopefully somewhat wiser.

The thing is, for all my beefy intentions, I never seem to make it. The biggest obstacle is size. To make a proper corned beef and cabbage dinner, you need to buy a whole corned beef, which weighs upward of 3 pounds, feeding at least eight. Usually on St. Patrick's Day I'm cooking for my tiny family of three, or two and a smidgen if you count what Dahlia eats of her dinner before clamoring for dessert.

This past year, however, I decided to try making a corned beef-cabbage-and-potato meal in a whole new way.

I had just written a *New York Times* article featuring the best baked potatoes I'd ever had, a variation on a Nigel Slater recipe. He stuffed his with pork rillettes and cheese. So I decided to try stuffing mine with slices of deli corned beef, which I hoped would add the same salty, savory kick as the rillettes but would be easier to find and possibly more apropos to serve on a day usually celebrated with pints of green beer.

[CONTINUED]

The dish was a success; even Dahlia ate it after she laboriously picked out the dill bits and tossed them from her tray in a green-black shower. I like this recipe better than your standard-issue boiled corned beef and cabbage dinner, and almost as much as corned beef on rye—an awfully hard morsel to beat.

4 russet potatoes (10 to 12 ounces each), scrubbed well

2 1/4 teaspoons kosher salt

3/4 pound thinly sliced corned beef, coarsely chopped

4 tablespoons (1/2 stick) unsalted butter, softened

1 tablespoon plus 1 teaspoon chopped fresh dill

Pinch freshly ground black pepper

1/4 cup grated Parmesan cheese

Serves 4

1. Preheat the oven to 425°F. Rub each potato with 1/2 teaspoon salt and pierce twice with a fork. Place the potatoes on a baking sheet and bake until the skin is crispy and the insides are tender when pierced with a fork, 1 hour to 70 minutes.

2. When the potatoes have cooled enough to handle, use a sharp knife to slice off the tops. Scoop out the insides, leaving about 1/4 inch attached to the skin, and transfer to a bowl. Add the corned beef, butter, dill, remaining salt, and pepper to the bowl and mash well with a fork.

3. Stuff the potato skins with the potato mixture. Divide the topping among the potatoes and sprinkle with the cheese. Return the potatoes to the oven and bake until heated through, about 10 minutes. Run under the broiler for an additional 1 to 2 minutes, until golden brown and the cheese has melted.

What Else?

- This basic method of rubbing the potatoes with salt and baking without foil, at relatively high heat, gives a very crisp-skinned potato that's ideal if you are the kind of person who likes to eat the potato skin. I certainly am, and this had become my standard baked potato method. Just make sure to use russet potatoes, which have a thicker and more crisp-able skin than thin-skinned red potatoes and Yukon Golds.

- When I make these for Daniel, I just skip the cheese and dust the top with a little flaky sea salt.

- Pastrami, a slice of coarse country pâté, leftover pot roast, and rillettes are all terrific substitutes for the corned beef if you are not serving this for St. Paddy's Day. Or if you've embraced rye bread as corned beef's one true soul mate and are happy to leave it at that.

CRISPY ROASTED CABBAGE

If a regular Irish boiled corned beef and cabbage dinner is the essence of soft, silky, and supple, my version is crisped, browned, crunchy—the cabbage included. Roasting it in slices gives the cabbage plenty of surface area to brown in the oven, while the center gets tender but doesn't turn soggy. We eat roasted cabbage all winter long and into spring, all the way up until the day the first asparagus show up at the farmers' market. Then we unceremoniously cast cabbage aside—until the next winter, when we are grateful for its hardy, sustaining, sweet presence in every market stall.

1 pound green cabbage (1 small or half a large one), cored
Olive or peanut oil, for brushing
Pinch kosher salt

Serves 4 to 6

Preheat the oven to 400°F. Cut the cabbage into 1-inch-thick slices. Brush the slices with olive or peanut oil and place on a rimmed baking sheet. Try to keep the pieces from falling apart (though if they do start to separate, that is okay). Sprinkle the cabbage with a generous seasoning of salt. Roast, turning once, until crispy and browned, 25 to 30 minutes.

What Else?

- Obviously you needn't limit yourself to serving this with corned beef. I like it as part of an all-vegetable meal, with brown rice and fried tofu croutons (see page 23). It's also lovely as a side dish for roast chicken, maybe under a dollop of sour cream or yogurt and showered with dill. Sometimes I make it by itself for lunch and eat it accompanied by toasted brown bread with plenty of butter. Sometimes I sprinkle grated cheese (pecorino is excellent) on top during the last 10 minutes of roasting. If you like cabbage, you will find plenty of ways to enjoy this simple dish.

WHOLE WHEAT IRISH SODA BREAD WITH RAISINS AND CARAWAY

On a trip to Dublin several years ago, I discovered that Irish soda bread in New York is nothing like Irish soda bread in Ireland.

In New York, Irish soda bread is packed with raisins and caraway, laden with sugar, and baked into a free-form round. It's so rich that dabbing on butter seems a profligate gesture, though I have to admit I do it anyway.

In Dublin, the Irish soda bread I sampled (also called Irish brown bread) was a more austere affair, delectable in a completely different way than its new-world kin. Baked in a loaf pan, it had a moist, cakey texture and wholemeal taste, but no dried fruit, spices, or sweetener kneaded into the mix. Spread with good, salted Irish butter as yellow as a baby chick and topped with marmalade or smoked salmon, it was a bready revelation, and I ate it as often as I could.

I thought about the distinct, pleasantly damp crumb and nutty flavor of that brown bread as I was trying to come up with a new recipe for Irish soda bread around St. Patrick's Day.

I wanted to keep the pockets of raisin chewiness and caraway tang of the New York soda breads I'd grown accustomed to, but I also wanted it to have more depth of toasty flavor like the Irish brown breads in Dublin. So I decided to cross the two recipes, pulling back on the sugar and adding some whole wheat flour to the mix while keeping the fruit and spice.

The result is just what I was hoping for: nutty and soft, with a deep rich flavor that is less sweet than your average scone, and a tender, biscuit-like texture that's best straight from the oven, or toasted if you've let it cool. Slather it with lots of salted yellow butter and dream about well-pulled Guinness, icy oysters, velvety salmon, and other Hibernian gustatory delights.

2 cups whole wheat pastry flour (see What Else?)

1 cup all-purpose flour

1/3 cup sugar

1 tablespoon baking powder

1 1/2 teaspoons kosher salt

1 teaspoon baking soda

1 1/2 cups plain whole milk yogurt

2 large eggs, lightly beaten

1/4 cup unsalted butter, melted

1 1/2 cups raisins

1 tablespoon caraway seeds

1. Preheat the oven to 350°F. Lightly grease a 10-inch round cake pan.
2. In a large bowl, combine the flours, sugar, baking powder, salt, and baking soda. In a separate bowl, whisk together the yogurt, eggs, and 2 tablespoons of the melted butter. Fold the wet ingredients into the dry until just combined, taking care not to overmix. Fold in the raisins and caraway seeds.
3. Scrape the dough out onto a lightly floured surface. Shape the dough into a round about 7 inches in diameter (it will spread to about 10 inches in diameter) and place it on the prepared cake pan. Score the round with a cross and drizzle with the remaining 2 tablespoons of melted butter. Bake until golden brown, 45 to 50 minutes. Serve warm if possible. Or toast slices before serving.

What Else?

*   There are some American versions of Irish soda breads laden with so much sugar and butter, anyone from Ireland would positively call them cake. This is not one of those recipes, though it's still sweeter and richer than what you'd get in Shannon. If you want it even sweeter, up the sugar to 1/2 or even 2/3 cup. For an even richer result, use sour cream in place of yogurt.

- You can bake this with all-purpose flour if you're not on a raise-the-fiber-content-in-your-diet quest as I am. I actually prefer the nutty flavor of whole wheat here, but I recognize that it might be an acquired taste.

- If you can't find whole wheat pastry flour, you can use regular whole wheat flour and expect a slightly heavier cake. Or add a little more all-purpose flour to the mix, using $1\frac{1}{2}$ cups all-purpose flour and $1\frac{1}{2}$ cups regular whole wheat flour.

- If you don't like caraway seeds, simply leave them out, or substitute cumin seeds, which will add a wacky and slightly Middle Eastern–inspired element to the mix.

- Teensy currants (Dahlia calls them baby raisins) are a nice substitute for the raisins.

OLIVE OIL–ALMOND CAKE WITH VANILLA MASCARPONE

What do you bring when you are invited to lunch at the house of a friend who pulls out all the stops when entertaining?

Where the meal is always truffled and foie gras–ed in every course; the wines are of fine, rare vintages; the cheeses raw; the meat perfectly cooked; and the setting at once pastoral and elegant as is possible within a one-hour drive of New York City?

Naturally, you bake a cake.

But not just any old cake. No, you bake the most fascinating, least expected, most ethereal cake you can think of.

In this case, I pulled out my tried-and-true recipe for olive oil–almond cake. This is one of my favorite recipes to bring somewhere for dinner. It's light, very moist, and intensely almond-y without resorting to almond extract, a rare feat in itself.

For these particular friends, I added a touch of buckwheat flour to the mix, which gave the final confection a nutty complexity and richness. Plus, even for a group of fantastic cooks and foodies who have been there, done that with almost every delightful comestible imaginable, I knew the chances of them having tried a buckwheat-olive oil–almond cake before were slim to none.

I can't say the cake stole the day, but it managed to delight and intrigue the other guests, and sate my own not-so-insignificant sweet tooth, not to mention hold its own against some mighty fine bottles of Chave Hermitage from the cellar. And that is good enough for me.

Serves 8 to 10

1/2 cup all-purpose flour
1/2 cup buckwheat flour
1/2 cup finely ground blanched almonds
1 1/2 teaspoons baking powder

1 teaspoon kosher salt

3 large eggs, lightly beaten

3/4 cup granulated sugar

1/2 cup extra-virgin olive oil

1/2 teaspoon vanilla extract

1 tablespoon freshly grated orange zest

1/2 cup freshly squeezed orange juice

1 vanilla bean, split in half lengthwise

2 cups mascarpone cheese

1 to 2 tablespoons confectioners' sugar, or more if you like
   it really sweet

1. Preheat the oven to 350°F. Grease and flour a 9-inch round cake pan or springform pan and set aside.

2. In a medium bowl, whisk together the all-purpose flour, buckwheat flour, ground almonds, baking powder, and salt to combine.

3. In the bowl of an electric mixer, whisk together the eggs and granulated sugar. Add the olive oil and whisk until the mixture is lighter in color and has thickened slightly. Whisk in the vanilla and orange zest, followed by the orange juice.

4. Add the dry ingredients to the bowl and fold them in by hand until thoroughly combined and no lumps remain.

5. Pour the batter into the prepared pan, and bake until the sides of the cake begin to pull away from the pan and a tester inserted into the middle comes out clean, 30 to 45 minutes.

6. Allow the cake to cool for 10 minutes in the pan, then gently remove it from the pan and allow it to cool completely on a rack.

7. To make the mascarpone cream, use the back of a knife to scrape the seeds out of the vanilla bean halves and put them into a bowl. Add the mascarpone and whisk until fluffy, then whisk in the confectioners' sugar. Serve dollops with the cake.

What Else?

- When I brought this to my friend's house, I iced it with brown butter frosting and decorated the top with candied, slivered almonds I had left over from some other recipe, though I can't for the life of me remember what. If you'd like to do some lily gilding, you can make the frosting by whisking confectioners' sugar and a little vanilla extract into brown butter until the butter is as thick as a runny icing or a custard sauce. Spoon it over the cake, letting it drip down the sides.

- If you aren't feeling the buckwheat flour, or if you don't have any on hand from blini making or what-have-you, you can substitute cornmeal (olive oil polenta cake is a classic), whole wheat pastry flour, or even regular all-purpose flour, which will give you the lightest cake.

- A fresh fruit compote is terrific with this cake. Use whatever fruit is in season, cook it down with a little sugar, honey, or maple syrup, and spoon it over the cake. The cranberry compote on page 339 works really well, and makes this Thanksgiving-perfect.

Spring

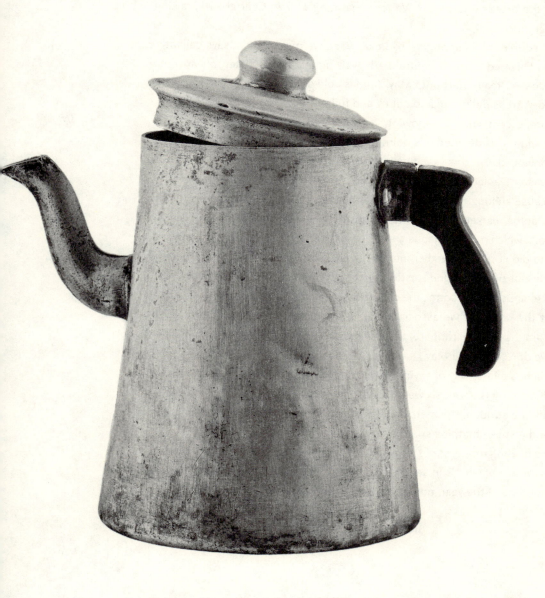

My husband swears that April is a winter month, and for most of our relationship, I've vehemently disagreed.

April is the month we met, I tell him; remember, the trees were blossoming and the breeze was warm? We took that long walk in Central Park, talking and laughing?

"Of course it was spring in my heart when we met," Daniel says gallantly. "But you shivered through Central Park, walking faster and faster to warm up. Spring doesn't really start until May. April is cold and nasty."

"No, April is delightful and balmy and full of sweet, sunny days."

"Sure, except when it's snowing. It always snows in April."

He and I have debated this point many times over the years, and I've never been convinced. But this year, finally, I had to concede.

It wasn't Daniel who finally convinced me. It was the farmers' market.

Because although the damp spring earth was finally pushing out tiny green threads, at the market, there still wasn't anything new to eat. April looked exactly like March, which mirrored January and February. True, the spinach was crisp and lively and didn't freeze together into an icy pile. The wintered-over leeks were finally dug out of the ground, tasting sweet and juicy. Errant bunches of herbs started to appear—the sorrel, the chives, maybe some early lovage.

But the real stuff we associate with spring—the ramps and the lettuces, the asparagus and the rhubarb, the tiny red strawberries bursting with juice— these we don't see until May.

Which is a long way of saying that when you're cooking seasonally in New York City, spring is about six weeks long—from early May to the end of June— when all of a sudden, the mercury shoots up, the roses bloom, the asparagus wilts, and just like that, it's summer.

This fleeting moment of spring is frantic and fantastic. There is an urgency to eat as much of what's in season as possible in a way that just doesn't apply any other time of the year, not even with August tomatoes.

First out of the gate is the asparagus. From the moment the skinny bunches start appearing at the market until our pores are saturated with their scent five weeks later, we eat asparagus as often as we can—at least four times a week, sometimes more.

Ditto ramps, those odoriferous alliums that look like floppy overgrown scallions and taste like sweet shallots dusted with lily. Ramps, which grow wild in marshy woodlands, are among the first greens to get pulled from the ground and rushed to the market. I can eat a whole mess of them just sautéed in butter, but they are even better as the base of a mussel stew (page 138) or tossed in a pan with asparagus and topped with fried eggs (page 141).

Other happy arrivals in the allium department include pale spring onions, the juicy, plump nascent incarnation of the mature, paper-swathed onions we take for granted all year long. There is nothing better sliced up into salads or caramelized with a little vinegar for a fresh-tasting agrodolce sauce to top seared fish (page 132). Then there are the tiny white stalks of green garlic that pop out in June. I've waited all winter for these, grumpily putting up with sprouted, dried, bruised garlic from the supermarket until the new crop comes in. And when it does, I celebrate by using the mild-tasting aromatic in absolutely anything I can get away with, rejoicing in the taut, fresh bulbs, which can be sliced up whole before they develop their thick outer husks.

I'm a little more judicious with spring rhubarb because it really does need a bucket of sugar to make it palatable, at least to me. I know there are people who adore its tart flavor with just a touch of honey, but I'm not one of them. I like my rhubarb sweet and mellow and preferably in the company of tiny garnet strawberries, either simmered into marmalade (page 158) or layered into a shortbread tart (page 155).

If I am going to decrease the sweetness when cooking with rhubarb, it's because I'm using it as a vegetable—which in fact it is. I like to think of savory rhubarb as being a little like lemon, but instead of clear thin juice, rhubarb has body. It makes a bracing, what-is-that-flavor sauce melted down almost all by itself for meats, fish, and, as tried on a whim, asparagus (page 143).

Another fleeting harbinger of spring is fiddlehead ferns, which I keep trying to develop a taste for.

I first saw them when I was seventeen and working at Dean & Deluca—back when there was just one Soho store and it only sold gourmet ingredients. The produce manager had brought in a sack full of the forest-foraged things. They were delicate, whirly, dark green discs covered in thin brown papery skin, and I thought they were beautiful. I was told to rub off the skin with a dish towel as if I were peeling roasted hazelnuts, then blanch the discs in salted water, blot dry, and cover with vinaigrette. I made them as soon as I got home.

Maybe my expectations were too high, but I thought they tasted like tree leaves.

Still, every April, when the snow melts and the air softens, my excitement rises as soon as I see fiddleheads piled in a basket. I know that once they show up, asparagus and strawberries can't be far behind, that winter is finally over.

And I always buy a small bag of the heralding ferns just to see if I've finally matured into appreciating them. So far, no go. But hope springs eternal.

APRIL

CREAMY LEEK GRATIN
WITH PARMESAN

For years, I thought those first, fat leeks to hit the farmers' market in April were newly grown spring leeks. It never occurred to me that they were actually left over from last year's crop. The farmers set aside a patch of leeks, cover them thickly with hay, and let them hibernate in the freezing ground all winter long, plucking them when the thaw comes. Wintered-over leeks get very sweet from this treatment, which is odd since I know I'd get very grumpy if you tried to do the same thing to me.

Leeks vinaigrette is usually my go-to dish when I want leeks to star. But this year, I got antsy and looked for another way to showcase the mild, earthy allium. After much careful consideration (as in, an idea popped into my head while I was unloading the dishwasher), I remembered the amazing, gooey, creamy leek gratin I'd sampled over at Franny's restaurant near my home. The sous-chef, Danny Amend, cooks up an elaborate creation, roasting the leeks in the wood oven before layering them into a casserole with heavy cream and cheese.

My version is streamlined and a bit lighter. I cut the cream with chicken broth and reduce the overall amount of cheese. It's rich without being heavy, and the leeks become wonderfully silky and deeply flavored as they slacken amidst all the bubbling cream, butter, and broth, crowned with a golden and crisp cheese topping.

I originally made this as a meatless main dish when my dairy-free husband Daniel was out of town, but it also makes a lovely side dish for something simple, maybe roasted chicken or broiled steak. And one night, I ate it piled on toasted multigrain bread for an odd but thoroughly satisfying dinner for one.

2 pounds leeks (4 to 5 medium), white and light green parts only,
    trimmed and halved lengthwise
1 cup chicken or vegetable stock

Serves 4 to 6

1 cup half-and-half or milk, plus additional as needed

3 tablespoons unsalted butter

3 tablespoons all-purpose flour

1/4 teaspoon kosher salt

1/8 teaspoon freshly ground black pepper

Pinch freshly grated nutmeg

Small pinch cayenne

1/2 pound Gruyère cheese, grated (about 2 cups)

2 ounces Parmesan cheese, grated (about 1/2 cup)

1. Preheat the oven to 400°F. Lightly grease a 9 × 13-inch baking pan.
2. Run the leeks under cool water to remove any grit between the layers. Bring a large pot of salted water to a boil. Simmer the leeks in the water until almost tender, about 10 minutes. Drain well and pat completely dry.
3. In a small saucepan, warm the stock and half-and-half or milk.
4. In a separate saucepan over medium-high heat, melt the butter. Add the flour and cook, stirring, until the roux is pale yellow and frothy, about 1 minute. Slowly whisk in the warm milk and stir until thickened, 2 to 3 minutes. Reduce the mixture to a simmer and season with salt, pepper, nutmeg, and cayenne; simmer 1 minute more. Whisk in the Gruyère until melted. If the mixture seems too thick, thin slightly with milk.
5. Transfer the leeks, cut-side up, to the prepared pan. Spoon the sauce over the leeks. Sprinkle the top with the Parmesan. Bake until the sauce is bubbling and golden, about 40 minutes.

What Else?

- There is no way to make this dish acceptable for people who, like Daniel, don't eat cheese and cream. I'll make it for myself when he's out of town, and then eat leftovers for lunch as long as it will last. I can also see bringing this to the kind of large, excessive family gathering where there is so much food anyone who is dairy-free wouldn't feel leek deprived. Or hungry.

[CONTINUED]

- You can prepare this gratin several hours ahead, right up to the baking step. Leave it assembled in the fridge until you are ready to bake, then pop it in the oven just before you want to serve it. I've also baked this ahead and reheated it with some success. It's still got a great flavor, but be careful to use low heat because the cheese in the sauce can get grainy if you use too high a heat. A 300°F oven for 20 to 30 minutes should do it.

POT-ROASTED LAMB
WITH MEYER LEMON

Here's the sad truth about pot roast. No matter how lovingly, how carefully, how masterfully it's coddled when cooked, if you start out with brisket, it always ends up stringy and dry.

The reason for this, I've recently learned, is that pretty much all of the brisket on offer is a very lean piece called "first cut" or "flat cut" brisket. And with leanness comes dryness. I've heard rumors that there exists another, better-tasting, fattier morsel of brisket called the second cut, but I've yet to meet one in the flesh.

Which means, when an occasion demands pot roast or bust (Passover, for example), I skip the brisket altogether and nestle another cut of fatty, flavorful meat into the pot. Usually, it's flanken or short ribs.

But last Passover I decided on a more experimental route. I bought a hunk of lamb shoulder, thinking I'd braise it à la my mother's pot roast, with lemon juice and garlic. (Even my mother has finally given up on brisket; she's a boneless short ribs convert, and her pot roast is all the better for it.)

I knew the lamb-lemon-garlic flavors would work well together—the combination is about as traditional in the Mediterranean as bagels and lox is in Brooklyn. And I figured lamb shoulder would take well to pot roasting. Since it is shot through with collagen and fat, which melt to moisten the meat during the long, slow stint in the oven, braising (which is what pot roasting is) is in fact its ideal cooking method.

Then came the wild card: A display of Meyer lemons caught my eye as I was prowling the greengrocer in search of a pomegranate to plunder (the seeds make a gorgeous garnish; see What Else?). I didn't find a pomegranate, but I bought several Meyer lemons to use in the braising liquid. They would be sweeter than their common cousins, but that sounded good to me.

And do you know what? It was good—very, very good. The lamb shoulder

[CONTINUED]

cooked up tender and spoonable, imbued with garlic and sweet-tart Meyer lemons, which made a thin but very flavorful pan sauce that tasted a little like marmalade, in a lovely, lamb-y, gamy way. The recipe added another chapter to the family pot roast chronicles, which I'm hopeful will continue apace for many years to come.

Serves 10 to 12

5 garlic cloves
1 tablespoon plus 1 pinch kosher salt
1 (3 1/2- to 4-pound) boneless lamb shoulder roast, untied
1 1/4 teaspoons freshly ground black pepper
2 Meyer lemons
1/3 cup olive oil

1. Mince 2 garlic cloves. Using a mortar and pestle or the flat side of a heavy knife, pound or mash the minced garlic with a pinch of salt until it turns to a paste.

2. Season the lamb all over with the salt and pepper and rub the garlic paste into the meat. Place the lamb in a large bowl or pan, cover tightly with plastic wrap, and refrigerate for at least 2 hours or overnight. Let the meat come to room temperature for 1 hour before cooking it.

3. When you're ready to cook the lamb, preheat the oven to 325°F. Finely grate the zest of both lemons and reserve; juice the lemons.

4. Heat the oil in a large Dutch oven until almost smoking. Sear the lamb in the oil until browned on all sides, about 10 minutes. Pour the lemon juice over the lamb and add enough water to come halfway up the sides of the meat (about 2 cups). Bring the liquid to a boil over high heat.

5. Cover the pot, transfer to the oven, and cook for 45 minutes. Meanwhile, mince the remaining 3 garlic cloves. Turn the meat over in the pot and add the garlic. Cover and cook 15 minutes longer. Then stir in the reserved lemon zest and continue to cook, uncovered, 15 minutes longer.

6. Remove from the oven and let stand 10 minutes before slicing and serving, with the pan juices spooned over the meat. Or, if you want to degrease this sauce, let the braise cool, spoon the grease from the top, then reheat and

serve. If you've got time, make this the day before, chill it overnight so the fat hardens on top of the sauce, then spoon it off before reheating.

What Else?

- If you don't have Meyer lemons around, regular lemons will do nicely. Or use a combination of 1 lemon and 1 tangerine. This will give you a flavor quite close to a Meyer lemon.

- If you can find pomegranate seeds, they make a stunning garnish. Or, if you're feeling a little more ambitious, make a pomegranate gremolata by combining the seeds with some minced garlic, grated lemon zest, and chopped parsley. Sprinkle it over slices of the roast when you serve it.

- A couple of anchovies thrown into the pot adds a certain ocean-ish je ne sais quoi.

- I love this recipe with short ribs or flanken (which is short ribs cut across the bone rather than with the bone). Anytime you cook meat on the bone, you get a lot more flavor. Plus the sauce gets terrific body from the marrow.

- If you want to make this with a regular beef brisket, go ahead. Just don't blame me if it's dry.

- If you substitute chicken broth for the water, you'll end up with a richer sauce. I never bother doing this because I like the clean lemony taste to stand alone, but it's a good option if you're looking for a more classic gravy flavor.

CURRIED COCONUT TOMATO SOUP

A play on cream of tomato soup, this recipe is supremely satisfying for the dairy-avoidant set (in other words, I can feed this to my husband).

It's just the thing to serve on those raw April days when it feels like March outside the door. Since this soup doesn't rely on any fresh produce, barring an onion and a little green garnish, you could even make it in winter, where it would be as welcome as the first warm breezes of spring.

The curry powder, boosted with coriander and cumin, adds an earthy, fragrant note that you definitely don't find in a can of Campbell's, and the coconut milk makes the whole thing ever so slightly sweet. It's a thinner, more brothy soup than the cream-based cream of tomato soups you usually find. But I like it all the better for this because I can eat more of it before filling up. It's got a flavor you won't want to end at the bottom of just one bowl.

Serves 2 to 4

2 tablespoons unsalted butter
1 Spanish onion, thinly sliced
1½ teaspoons kosher salt, plus additional to taste
1½ teaspoons curry powder
½ teaspoon ground coriander
½ teaspoon ground cumin
Pinch chili powder
1 (28-ounce) can diced or whole peeled plum tomatoes
2 (13.5-ounce) cans coconut milk
Chopped fresh cilantro, mint, or basil, for garnish

1. In a large saucepan over medium heat, melt the butter. Add the onion and ½ teaspoon salt. Reduce the heat to medium-low, cover, and cook, stirring occasionally, until the onion is meltingly tender, about 15 minutes. Lower the

heat and add a sprinkle of water if necessary to keep the onion from browning.

2. Stir in the curry powder, coriander, cumin, and chili powder, and cook for 1 minute. Stir in the tomatoes and their juice and 4 cups water. Bring the mixture to a simmer over medium-high heat. Simmer, uncovered, for 20 minutes.

3. Working in batches, transfer the soup to a blender and puree until smooth. Return the soup to the pan. Whisk in 1 can coconut milk. Spoon off 1/2 cup cream from the top of the second can (reserve the remaining milk for another use, such as coconut rice, page 49) and whisk it into the soup. Stir in the remaining 1 teaspoon salt. Gently heat the soup over medium-low heat for 10 minutes, or until it reaches the desired consistency. Ladle the soup into bowls and garnish with cilantro.

What Else?

- I've been meaning to try this with cream instead of coconut milk when Daniel isn't around, but I haven't gotten around to it yet. If you are tempted, try using about 2 cups of cream or half-and-half in place of the coconut milk. And please let me know how it turns out.

- If case you've been wondering what the difference is between "lite" coconut milk and regular coconut milk, the "lite" stuff has water added to it (and sometimes additives such as gums to make it thicker). I say avoid it, and if you want a lighter coconut milk, just add water to the regular stuff. It will end up being cheaper and better tasting.

- Toasted coconut chips, stirred together with a little flaky sea salt, make a great topping for this soup if you want something crunchy. Or try serving it with the paratha on page 278 if you are feeling ambitious. The paratha comes together quickly (20 to 30 minutes) and you can do it while the soup simmers.

[CONTINUED]

- For a richer soup that's a bit more complex and a bit less tomatoey, substitute chicken or vegetable stock for the water.

- To turn this into a full meal, add a few handfuls of small peeled shrimp, fish chunks, or bay scallops to the soup during the last 5 minutes of cooking, and serve with rice or paratha (page 278).

SAVORY MATZO BREI WITH BLACK PEPPER AND HONEY

There are the sweet-toothed people of the world, and there are those who like it salty. For most of the year, the divide goes like this: bread pudding or blood pudding; chocolate chips or potato chips; honey-roasted peanuts or roasted with salt. But for Jews during Passover, the dichotomy is reduced into one telling choice: How do you take your matzo brei, savory or sweet?

Growing up, the brei—rhymes with *fry*—was always savory. Made from matzo fried hard and crisp with eggs, salt, pepper, and occasionally onions, it was crunchy, browned around the edges, and as salty as bacon (which we joked about adding but never worked up the nerve to try). The recipe was so ingrained in our family's psyche that, as a child, I didn't even realize there was another way to make it.

Then my sister came home for Passover during her first year at the University of Michigan and poured maple syrup over her brei. Syrup on matzo brei? Had I known this was a possibility, I would have explored it much earlier, given my penchant for things sweet and gooey. A whole new world opened up—matzo brei with honey, cinnamon sugar, brown sugar, confectioners' sugar—let's just say lots of sugar.

Still, no matter how much I experimented with sweet toppings, the lure of my parents' matzo brei with plenty of brown sautéed onions, loads of black pepper, and a heady dose of nostalgia was too strong to ignore. Although I am a committed member of the sweet-toothed tribe, when it comes to matzo brei, I go both ways.

This recipe is a perfect illustration of having my salt with frosting on top. It's mostly savory, from black pepper and a jolt of salt. But the honey drizzle at the end pays homage to matzo brei's sweet potential . . . and my own ambivalent inclinations.

4 matzo squares, broken into large pieces

4 large eggs

2 tablespoons whole milk

1/2 teaspoon kosher salt

1/2 teaspoon freshly ground black pepper, plus additional for garnish

6 tablespoons unsalted butter

Coarse sea salt, for sprinkling

Honey, for drizzling

Serves 2

1. Place the matzo in a large bowl and cover with warm water. Soak until slightly pliable but still firm, 1 to 2 minutes; drain well.

2. In a separate bowl, whisk together the eggs, milk, salt, and 1/2 teaspoon pepper. Stir in the matzo.

3. In a large skillet, melt the butter over high heat. When the foam subsides, stir in the egg-matzo mixture. Scramble the mixture with a spatula for a minute, then pat into the bottom of the pan and cook, without moving, until golden brown on the bottom, 2 to 3 minutes. Flip the matzo brei in chunks (it's okay if it looks a little messy). Scramble it around, pressing down with the spatula. Cook until it has a fluffy center and crisp edges, about 1 minute.

4. Transfer the matzo brei to serving plates. Sprinkle with sea salt and black pepper; drizzle with honey.

What Else?

- If you want to try the oniony matzo brei of my childhood, skip the honey, and top the brei with onions cooked in butter and a pinch of salt until very dark brown. You can follow the recipe for browned onions on page 51 if you like.

- If you like sweeter matzo brei, reduce the salt to $1/4$ teaspoon, skip the pepper, and pour on the honey, or maple syrup if that's your fancy.

- I've made this with whole wheat matzos, and it's a sad, heavy affair. If you do want to up the fiber content, you can try this with 1 whole wheat matzo and 3 regular ones. Egg matzo or egg and onion matzo also work well if that's what you've got.

GREEN-POACHED EGGS WITH SPINACH AND CHIVES

I call this creation "green eggs no ham," and it's an ideal vegetarian dish. Spiked with lemon zest, chives, chile, and cream, it really doesn't want bacon or ham or all the other meaty things I automatically think of when I think of eggs.

It's based on a recipe for sorrel poached eggs that I came up with when I used to have a sorrel plant on my deck. The poor plant succumbed to the squirrels, who used it to bury (and aggressively dig up) nuts. Although I can certainly buy sorrel at the farmers' market, it's not dependably available.

Spinach, however, is always there except in the broiling heat of summer. From September to June, I can count on finding bunches of the crinkly, dark green leaves, ready to be tossed into salads or wilted in a pan of butter or olive oil, and sometimes crowned with runny eggs. I like this for supper (not dinner; eggs are for supper), but it's also excellent for brunch.

2 tablespoons unsalted butter

Serves 4

3 fat scallions, sliced (white and light greens separated
    from dark greens)

1 garlic clove, finely chopped

1/3 cup finely chopped fresh chives

10 ounces fresh baby spinach (about 4 quarts)

1/4 teaspoon kosher salt, plus additional for seasoning

Freshly ground black pepper to taste

1/3 cup heavy cream

Finely grated zest of 1 lemon

4 large eggs

Chile flakes (such as Aleppo, Urfa, or crushed red), for serving

Coarse sea salt, for serving

Buttered toast, for serving

1. Melt the butter in a large skillet over medium-high heat until the foam subsides. Add the white and light green scallions and garlic and cook, stirring, until fragrant, about 30 seconds. Stir in the chives. Toss in the spinach, a handful at a time, letting each batch wilt slightly before adding more. Add 1/4 teaspoon salt and black pepper. Stir in the cream and lemon zest; let simmer until the spinach is very soft, about 3 minutes.

2. Using the back of a spoon, make 4 little indentations in the spinach—think of them as nests for the eggs. Crack the eggs into the nests. Lower the heat to medium-low and sprinkle the eggs with salt and pepper. Cover the pan and let the eggs cook until almost opaque, about 3 minutes. Turn off the heat and let the eggs rest, covered, until done to taste, 30 seconds for yolks that are runny (whites should be completely cooked through), or longer if you like harder eggs.

3. Carefully scoop the eggs and greens into two bowls. Season each bowl with chile flakes and flaky salt; garnish them with scallion greens. Serve with buttered toast.

What Else?

- If you want to try this with sorrel, simply substitute it for the spinach. It will break down into more of a sauce than the spinach does, and the color will fade from verdant to olive drab, but the flavor will pop. Leave out the lemon zest when using sorrel; you won't need it.

- If you are looking for a simple spinach side dish, skip the eggs and serve this as creamed spinach.

- Naturally, when Daniel is around, I will make this without the cream. I just leave it out and add an extra chunk of butter (yes, he can eat butter, just not cream, milk, or cheese).

VIETNAMESE GRILLED STEAK AND CABBAGE SALAD WITH PEANUTS, MINT, AND CHILES

By the time April rolls around, I'm ready to be done with cabbage. It's not that I don't appreciate its stalwart, pale presence at the otherwise near-depleted farmers' market of winter. I do. But after months and months of the stuff, you can bet I've sautéed, stewed, fried, and roasted the orb to the outer limits of my cruciferous desires.

That's when I know it's time for a new recipe, something slightly out of my Eastern European comfort zone, to whet my appetite and get me back into a cabbage groove.

Whenever I start to get that winter palate fatigue, my best cure is usually a dish inspired by more temperate climes, places rich with spunky spice and heat and plenty of lively citrus.

My first thought was to take a mental trip to Mexico and whip up some fish tacos piled high with a cilantro-spiked cabbage slaw. I kept daydreaming, and the combination of cilantro, cabbage, and lime juice made my mind skip over to a place I've been to in restaurants only: Vietnam. I remembered a cabbage salad spiked with chile, garlic, fish sauce, limes, and herbs that I often order, and immediately sat down to scour the Internet trying to find it.

There were hundreds of renditions, some with meat, some without. Since I was looking for dinner, I cherry-picked from the selections, adding and subtracting ingredients to match what I had in the fridge and freezer (namely, a flank steak), and what I could easily pick up at the store around the corner (ginger, lime, cilantro, but not lemongrass).

I made a pungent marinade for the steak, and while it marinated I whisked together a vibrant soy sauce–based vinaigrette and tossed it with the shredded cabbage. The dressing was so bright and flavorful it immediately made me overcome any cabbage inhibitions, and I inhaled half the bowl before I remembered that there was also some nice slices of bloody steak on my plate, too.

It was a perfect winter-doldrums meal that made spring seem not so very far away after all.

Serves 4

¹/₄ cup soy sauce

Freshly squeezed juice and finely grated zest of 1 lime

2 tablespoons grated fresh gingerroot

2 teaspoons toasted (Asian) sesame oil

2 garlic cloves, finely chopped

1¹/₄-pound flank steak, rinsed and patted dry

2 carrots, peeled and trimmed

10 cups shredded napa or regular cabbage (about ¹/₂ head)

¹/₄ cup chopped fresh cilantro (or use mint or basil)

Kosher salt and freshly ground black pepper

2 tablespoons chopped peanuts (optional)

FOR THE SPICY VINAIGRETTE

2 tablespoons soy sauce

1 tablespoon rice wine vinegar

2 tablespoons extra-virgin olive or peanut oil

1 teaspoon Thai or Vietnamese fish sauce, such as or nam pla or nuoc mam

Freshly squeezed juice of 1 lime

Pinch cayenne

1 garlic clove, finely chopped

1. Whisk together the soy sauce, lime juice and zest, gingerroot, and sesame oil. With a mortar and pestle or with the flat side of a knife, mash the garlic into a paste. Whisk into the marinade. Place the steak in a shallow dish and cover with the marinade, turning completely to coat. Cover the dish with plastic wrap and refrigerate for at least 1 hour and up to 12. Remove the steak from the refrigerator 30 minutes prior to cooking.

2. In a food processor fitted with the large grating attachment, shred the carrots. Turn them out into a large bowl. Add the cabbage and cilantro. Cover and toss well. Cover tightly with plastic wrap and refrigerate for up to 3 hours.

[CONTINUED]

3. To make the vinaigrette, in a small bowl, whisk together the soy sauce, vinegar, olive or peanut oil, fish sauce, lime juice, and cayenne. Using a mortar and pestle or with the back of a knife, mash the garlic to a paste; whisk into the vinaigrette.

4. Preheat the broiler and position a rack in the top third of the oven. Remove the steak from the marinade, scraping off any excess, and season with salt and pepper. Transfer the steak to a baking sheet. Broil, turning once halfway through, until browned, about 3 minutes per side for medium-rare. Transfer the steak to a cutting board and let rest for 5 minutes. Thinly slice the steak against the grain.

5. To assemble, add just enough of the vinaigrette to the salad to coat it and toss well. Taste and add more dressing or salt or lime juice if desired. Place the salad onto the center of a platter and top with the steak. Sprinkle with the chopped peanuts, if desired, drizzle with more vinaigrette, and serve.

What Else?

- If you're absolutely done with cabbage but crave a tangy, meaty hunk of flesh, make the steak and marinade part of this dish and serve it by itself, or on a bed of watercress or arugula.

- The steak is a great recipe for summer grilling season, too. Serve it with sliced heirloom tomatoes and/or cucumbers if you can get nice ones.

- If you love mango, add some ripe cubes to the cabbage salad; it gives it an amazing sweet burst of flavor.

- This makes a light meal; if you want to add a hefty carb, I would recommend either plain rice or coconut brown rice (page 49), which isn't traditional but the flavors work nicely together.

ROASTED CHICKEN LEGS WITH SMOKED PAPRIKA, BLOOD ORANGE, AND GINGER

Of all the chicken parts a person can cook up for dinner, my number one choice is bone-in, succulent thighs. I suppose if I could easily buy a package of chicken necks and tails at the supermarket I might grab those instead. But since I can't, I don't, and I reach for thighs every time I want a quick-cooking poultry dinner.

Over the years I think I've flavored chicken thighs in nearly every possible way. The rule is, slather them with salt, garlic (de rigueur), and any other seasonings I can find in my pantry and fridge, then broil or roast until the skin is speckled brown and crisp and the meat juices run clear. I rarely make the same roasted chicken thighs dish twice and almost never write down the recipe, creating something new every time I unwrap the package.

But these particular thighs were worth repeating. There is something about the combination of orange zest, smoked paprika, cilantro, ginger, and garlic that is brawny, spicy, zippy, and utterly appealing, so I jotted down the recipe before I could forget it. I used the last of the season's blood oranges, but regular oranges are perfectly fine.

And I imagine the same savory flavors would work well with chicken necks and tails, too, should you be lucky enough to have them on hand.

Serves 4

¼ cup freshly squeezed orange juice, preferably blood orange

2 tablespoons extra-virgin olive oil

3 garlic cloves, finely chopped

2 tablespoons cilantro leaves, plus additional for garnish

1 small jalapeño, seeded if desired, and chopped

1 tablespoon grated fresh gingerroot

1¼ teaspoons kosher salt

[CONTINUED]

1 teaspoon freshly grated orange zest

3/4 teaspoon smoked hot paprika

2 1/2 pounds bone-in, skin-on chicken thighs and drumsticks,
    rinsed and patted dry

Sliced scallions, for serving

Orange wedges, for serving

1. In a blender, combine the orange juice, oil, garlic, cilantro, jalapeño, ginger, salt, orange zest, and paprika and blend until the garlic and jalapeño are pureed.

2. Combine the chicken and marinade in a large bowl. Cover with plastic wrap and transfer to the refrigerator to marinate for at least 1 hour (or overnight if you can plan that far ahead).

3. When you are ready to cook the chicken, preheat the oven to 475°F. Line a large baking sheet with aluminum foil and top with the chicken. Roast, turning once, until the chicken skin is golden and the meat juices are no longer pink, about 40 minutes. Serve, sprinkled with scallions and cilantro, with orange wedges for squeezing over the meat.

What Else?

- This dish is spicy. Not in a burn-your-mouth, gulp-water kind of way, but in a slow-building-burn manner. So proceed with caution when debating whether or not to add the jalapeño seeds. Even without them, it's fiery hot. With them, it's incendiary. If you'd rather downplay the heat, use sweet paprika rather than hot smoked paprika.

- Regular paprika works, too, but the flavor won't have that smoky edge.

- This dish has a lot of ingredients for a weeknight dinner, but most of them are staples, at least in my house. If you don't have something, you can probably leave it out. The combination might not be quite as transcendent without, say, the ginger or the jalapeño. But I promise it will still be good enough to eat.

- This goes really nicely with the bulgur "pilaf" on page 120, the barley on page 125, or the quinoa on page 150. Polenta would be lovely as well.

BULGUR "PILAF" WITH SWISS CHARD AND DRIED APRICOTS

When I think of pilaf, I think of Istanbul, where Daniel and I spent a delayed honeymoon six months after we were married. The whole city was magical, especially the food, which I remember as spice-filled, nut-speckled, rose water–drizzled morsels of heaven.

One of the most distinct and memorable dishes was one we sampled at the house of a friend of a friend. Engin Akin, an expert on Ottoman palace cuisine and a crackerjack cook, invited us over for a historic meal inspired by what the sultans ate during Ottoman times. I was expecting to be awed by the food but I did not expect my favorite dish to be a humble bulgur pilaf, which seemed more peasant than royal. Ms. Akin quickly set me straight.

"The Ottomans ate bulgur in pilaf and in soups at Topkapi Palace," she said, spooning me out a portion laced with pumpkin and chickpeas.

It looked plain and brown, but the flavors exploded on my tongue—hints of cinnamon, allspice, and plenty of butter. It was so good that I immediately understood why a sultan who could command dishes from anywhere in his far-flung empire would insist on bulgur.

This pilaf is inspired by those exotic yet homey flavors. Since I don't cook the grain with sautéed onions and stock, I don't know that it can technically be called pilaf (hence the quotation marks). But recently, I've been cooking bulgur with plenty of water, like pasta, which lets me simmer it until the grains are just tender but not mushy, and I don't have to worry about getting the amount of liquid perfect.

I added some tender shoots of Swiss chard that had finally made its way back to the farmers' market to give the dish some color and a vegetable quotient, along with dried apricots for sweetness and pistachios for crunch. Overall it's a heartier, more filling, and less nuanced dish than the one Ms. Akin served me, but no less compelling for the lack of authenticity.

1 cup bulgur

1 cinnamon stick

1/2 cup dried apricots, cut into 1/4-inch cubes

1 1/2 tablespoons unsalted butter

1/2 cup roughly chopped raw pistachios

3/4 teaspoon ground cumin

1/2 teaspoon kosher salt

1 tablespoon extra-virgin olive oil

2 garlic cloves, finely chopped

1 shallot, finely chopped

1 bunch Swiss chard, stems removed and leaves chopped

1/4 teaspoon freshly ground black pepper

Freshly squeezed lemon juice or pomegranate molasses,
    for drizzling

1. Bring a large pot of salted water to a boil. Add the bulgur and cinnamon; cook for about 9 minutes. Stir in the apricots and cook 2 to 3 minutes more, or until the bulgur is tender (this might vary depending on how coarse the bulgur is). Drain well and discard the cinnamon.

2. In a large skillet over medium-high heat, melt the butter. Add the pistachios, cumin, and 1/4 teaspoon salt. Cook, stirring, until golden, about 2 minutes. Transfer to a bowl.

3. Wipe out the skillet with a paper towel. Return it to medium heat and add the oil, garlic, and shallot. Cook, stirring, until the garlic is fragrant, about 30 seconds. Add the chard, the remaining 1/4 teaspoon salt, and the pepper. Cook, tossing, until the chard is wilted, about 3 minutes. Stir in the bulgur mixture and pistachios. Toss over the heat for 1 minute until warmed through. Transfer to serving plates and drizzle with lemon juice or pomegranate molasses.

What Else?

- Spinach makes a good Swiss chard stand-in. Use 1 large bunch or 1 quart baby spinach. I've also made this with kale, and it's delicious, but the kale needs a few extra minutes in the skillet to soften properly. If it's still tough after 5 minutes, stir in a few tablespoons of water to help steam it.

- Slivered almonds or pine nuts can be substituted for the pistachios, and you can use practically any dried fruit in place of the apricot. Raisins, prunes, and cranberries will work particularly well.

- If you were in Turkey, you might find a similar dish drizzled with brown butter. If this sounds good to you, by all means go for it. I've done it many times and it's divine, if on the rich side of pilaf. That's not a bad thing, as long as you know what you're getting.

- If you fry an egg or two and slide them on top of this pilaf, it will stand as a meal all by itself.

A Dish by Another Name

- To make Quinoa "Pilaf" with Swiss Chard and Dried Apricots, replace the bulgur with quinoa and cook for 8 minutes. It still won't be a classic pilaf, but you won't have to worry about the grains overcooking and turning mushy.

QUICK-BRAISED PORK CHOPS WITH SPRING GREENS AND ANCHOVIES

While winter demands long-simmered stews of Neanderthal-size meat hunks, springtime calls for quicker, more gentle braises of smaller cuts of meat. Pork chops are perfect. They take under thirty minutes to cook, but have the warming, rich flavor you want when those April showers beat down on the windows and the blustery raw wind rattles the glass.

I've kept things pretty minimal in this recipe, searing the chops until well bronzed, then adding butter, shallot, anchovies, and a little chicken broth for a deeply flavored pan sauce. But the bitter, tangy arugula is really what makes this dish scream "spring!" It adds just the right zesty note to contrast with the porkiness of the chops. We ate this dish with scallion and carrot-flecked barley (page 125) and it was a lovely match. But polenta will make you happy, too.

Serves 2

2 center-cut bone-in pork chops, about 1 1/2 inches thick
Kosher salt and freshly ground black pepper,
    for seasoning
2 tablespoons extra-virgin olive oil
2 tablespoons unsalted butter
2 tablespoons finely chopped shallot
3 anchovy fillets, finely chopped
1/4 cup chicken stock
1 large bunch arugula, stems trimmed (about 5 ounces)

1. Season the pork chops with salt and pepper. Heat the oil to shimmering in a large skillet over medium-high heat. Add the pork chops and sear, without moving, until dark golden, 2 to 3 minutes per side. Transfer the chops to a plate.

[CONTINUED]

2. Return the skillet to the stove and reduce the heat to medium. Melt the butter in the pan. Add the shallot and anchovies; cook, stirring, 1 minute. Pour in the stock. Toss in the arugula, coating it lightly with the pan sauce. Nestle the pork chops on top of the arugula. Cover and braise over low heat until the pork chops are just cooked through, about 15 minutes.

What Else?

- Tracking down really thick pork chops can be hard because they're not the kind of thing sitting in the supermarket meat case, waiting to be your dinner. Meat farmers at the market sometimes have them, and any butcher will cut them for you, however, but if the supermarket is your only option, you can use thinner chops. Just adjust the cooking time so they don't overbake and toughen. For 1-inch chops, start checking after 10 minutes; for 1/2-inch chops, after 5.

- If you can get pea shoots, they make a fantastic and unexpected substitute for the arugula.

- If you don't like anchovies . . . add them anyway. You really don't taste them here, but they just add a layer of richness and complexity that really makes this dish special. That said, I won't be mad if you substitute 1/4 cup chopped olives or a couple of tablespoons capers instead.

BARLEY WITH CARROTS, SCALLIONS, AND MAYBE PARMESAN

Cooking shredded carrots along with soft, nubby barley grains is a great way to get your toddler to eat vegetables. Or at least it's a relatively reliable way to get my toddler to do so. Of course when it comes to feeding a certain two-year-old, it's always a gamble. In any case, Daniel and I dependably like the gentle, moist barley seasoned with sharp spring scallions and plenty of good olive oil. So even if Dahlia turns up her nose, this dish will find a welcoming plate.

It's good with hearty braised meats such as the pork chop with greens (page 123), or any kind of flesh you've got stewing. And I also like it very much with crisp-skinned broiled or roasted chicken, such as the gingery, paprika-scented thighs on page 117.

Serves 2 to 4

1 cup barley
2 medium carrots, trimmed, peeled, and grated
1/3 cup finely grated Parmesan cheese (optional)
2 tablespoons extra-virgin olive oil
2 scallions, white and light green parts, thinly sliced
1/4 teaspoon kosher salt
1/4 teaspoon freshly ground black pepper

1. Bring a large pot of salted water to a boil. Add the barley; reduce the heat and simmer until almost tender, 50 to 60 minutes. Stir in the carrots and cook until the carrots are tender and the grains are completely cooked, 5 to 10 minutes longer.
2. Drain well and transfer the mixture to a large bowl. Stir in the remaining ingredients; serve warm.

What Else?

- The cooking time for barley varies widely, I've found, so you will have to keep checking it. If the water level gets too low before the barley is done, you can add more hot water as needed. It's better to start out with a lot because you will be draining off any excess at the end, pasta style, anyway,

- The cheese is strictly optional here. I like it, but you-know-who prefers it without. You can also stir the cheese into your own portion just before serving.

- Sometimes I stir in a pasted garlic clove to give this more oompf. It's also good served with a squirt of Sriracha or other hot sauce, though what isn't?

A Dish by Another Name

- For Farro with Carrots, Scallions, and Parmesan, simply substitute farro for the barley. The cooking time might be different. Some types of farro cook in 20 minutes while some take an hour. Just follow the time frame on the farro package (if it has one), otherwise keep tasting it. It's ready when the grain is tender, but the hull won't necessarily split.

COCONUT FUDGE BROWNIES

Dense and chewy, these brownies are closer to chocolate truffles or a bowl of ganache frosting than they are to crumbly little cakes. The coconut oil gives them more chew than even the moistest usual recipe and a flavor that's as tasty as a Mounds bar. They don't cut as neatly as cakey brownies but their intense fudge flavor more than makes up for their messy appearance (or at least I think so).

Whatever you do, don't overbake these. You want them just on the solid side of chocolate sauce. Overbaking destroys their charms. As my friend Robin said when she accidentally overbaked a batch, "They taste like Passover brownies." Which is not a good thing. And if you do underbake them slightly and they run when you cut them, pretend you meant them to be like that all along (and serve them with a spoon).

"Do you like my molten chocolate brownies?" you can ask your friends. I promise you, they will.

Makes about 24 brownies

1/3 cup cocoa powder

1/2 cup plus 2 tablespoons boiling water

2 ounces unsweetened chocolate, finely chopped

4 tablespoons unsalted butter, melted

1/2 cup plus 2 tablespoons coconut oil

2 large eggs

2 large egg yolks

2 teaspoons vanilla extract

2 1/2 cups sugar

1 3/4 cups all-purpose flour

3/4 teaspoon kosher salt

3 ounces bittersweet chocolate, cut into 1/2-inch pieces

2 cups sweetened shredded coconut

Fleur de sel, for sprinkling

[CONTINUED]

1. Preheat the oven to 350°F. Lightly grease a 9 × 13-inch baking pan.

2. In a large mixing bowl, whisk the cocoa powder and boiling water together until smooth. Add the unsweetened chocolate and whisk until the chocolate has melted. Whisk in the melted butter and coconut oil. (The mixture may look curdled.) Add the eggs, egg yolks, and vanilla, and continue to whisk until combined. Whisk in the sugar until fully incorporated. Add the flour and salt and fold with a spatula until just combined. Fold in the bittersweet chocolate pieces.

3. Scrape half the batter into the prepared pan and smooth it into an even layer with a spatula. Sprinkle 1 cup of the shredded coconut on top of the batter. Spread the remaining batter over the coconut. Top with a layer of the remaining 1 cup shredded coconut. Sprinkle with fleur de sel and bake until a tester inserted in the center of the brownie is just set and shiny, 30 to 35 minutes. If you test it with a toothpick, it will seem wet, but that's okay. It solidifies as it cools. Transfer the pan to a wire rack to cool completely before cutting into squares.

What Else?

- Don't try to substitute that unsweetened dessicated coconut you got in the health food store in place of the sweetened shreds from the supermarket. Unsweetened coconut will be too dry, and won't give you the melt-in-the-mouth texture of the sweetened, preservative-filled stuff (sad, but true . . .).

- If you don't have coconut oil, you can use all melted butter, or a combination of butter and peanut or safflower oil. It won't be as coconutty or as chewy but will still taste delightful.

- If you're a nutty kind of person, you can add toasted walnuts or almonds in place of half the coconut flakes.

- Tart dried cherries make a nice addition here. Fold in 1/2 cup along with the chopped chocolate.

A Dish by Another Name

- To make Olive Oil Brownies, substitute extra-virgin olive oil for the coconut oil and omit the shredded coconut. Or leave the coconut in and you'll get Coconut–Olive Oil Brownies.

MAY

PAN-ROASTED PACIFIC HALIBUT WITH SPRING ONIONS AND HONEY BALSAMIC

Contrary to what I thought for most of my life, spring onions are not just another name for the ubiquitous scallion. Spring onions are lovely, fleeting things, tender young alliums plucked from their earthy home while still slim and meek, before they have a chance to turn bulbous and fat, pungent and strong. (Scallions, for the record, are a different variety of allium altogether.)

As you'd think, spring onions appear in the farmers' market along with the other early crops—asparagus, strawberries, sugar snap peas—usually in early May. And when I see them, I pounce. They are so mild that I can slice a whole bunch without crying one single tear, whereas regular old onions reduce me to a saline puddle after the first few cuts.

You can use them as you would a regular onion, but they are so succulent, I like to highlight them rather than bury them in the base of a sauce or soup.

This recipe is a nice, simple way to take full advantage of their flavor and plump texture. I cook the onions gently with balsamic vinegar and a little honey to bring out their sweetness, then serve them with an equally gentle-flavored protein—in this case, seared Pacific halibut—though nearly any mild, white-fleshed fish would work.

4 Pacific halibut fillets (about 8 ounces each), rinsed and patted dry

Freshly ground black pepper

3 bunches spring onions

6 tablespoons extra-virgin olive oil

6 thyme sprigs, plus leaves for garnish

Kosher salt or coarse sea salt

6 tablespoons balsamic vinegar, more for serving

2 teaspoons honey

Chopped fresh chives, for garnish

Serves 4

1. Season the fish with black pepper. Trim the spring onions, including the hairy bottoms, but leave the root end intact; remove the outer layer. Cut the onions into quarters.

2. In a very large sauté pan, heat 2 tablespoons oil over medium heat. Add the onions and thyme and season lightly with salt and pepper. Cover and cook until almost tender, about 3 minutes.

3. Uncover the pan, carefully turn the onions, and continue to cook until they caramelize, about 3 minutes more. Add 2 tablespoons of the balsamic vinegar and the honey to the pan, let cook for 20 seconds, then immediately transfer the onions to a bowl.

4. Heat the remaining oil in the pan until very hot. Lower the heat to medium-low, add the fish, skin-side down, and cook until just opaque, about 4 minutes a side. Add the remaining balsamic vinegar and remove from the heat.

5. Transfer the fish to four serving plates and top each fillet with some onion mixture. Drizzle with additional vinegar if desired and sprinkle with salt. Garnish with the thyme leaves and chives.

What Else?

- The season for spring onions is very short, spanning from a few weeks to about a month before the greens fall off and the onions mature, their skins turning from moist to papery. If you miss it or can't find them, use the mildest, sweetest regular onions you can find, such as Vidalia, Walla Walla, or red onions.

- You can use any kind of fish here, as long as you adjust the cooking time if the fillets are thinner or thicker. Mackerel works really well, and it's become one of my favorite sustainable fish. You'll find tips on how to cook it on page 246. Sardines are another spot-on pairing (their dark meat loves the sweet-and-sour flavors of the onions), though you will probably want to grill rather than sauté them so the skin gets nice and crisp.

[CONTINUED]

- If you're not a fish lover, these sweet-tart onions are divine with almost any other protein—use them on top of grilled steaks or chicken, or pile them on a hamburger. They're also fantastic layered with fresh mozzarella and arugula on a ciabatta sandwich.

- I like to eat delicate spring onions raw and thinly sliced. Their amenable flavor isn't too sharp to savor in salads, tossed in a tangle of spring lettuces. I also love them as a condiment for grilled meats, drizzled with a little lemon juice and chili powder. Serve this with a steak or lamb chops, and your friends will wonder what your secret is.

- Chives are the first green, edible things to come up in the pots on my deck in spring, so I tend to use them with abandon while waiting for the thyme and mint to bounce back. And I like how they highlight the pungent, mustard, herbal taste of the onions. But any fresh green herb works here, so feel free to substitute your favorite. My second choice would be mint, followed by cilantro.

FRISÉE SALAD WITH
BACON AND EGGS

For years, the be-all and end-all of frisée salads was the one I fell in love with at the Odeon in Tribeca. I used to frequent the place in my prechild, going-out-on-the-town-days, back when it was one of the few late-night restaurants where you could get a full meal at 1:00 A.M. (now even typing this is making me tired). I'd pop in postdancing and ravenous, and order the frisée salad, which was comprised of a shower of plump, confited garlic cloves, a pig's worth of fried lardons, plenty of crunchy croutons, and a mound of blue cheese. Somewhere in the bowl were a few wilted frisée leaves, though to be honest I might have left them on the bottom of the bowl when I'd eaten my fill. This salad was not about dieting. It was about flavorful excess, and I adored it.

Fast-forward to my more restrained, grown-up version. I have since discovered that I actually like frisée, and so in my salad, I use enough of the pale, curly greens to actually contribute some wholesome vegetable matter to the mix. I skipped the caramelized garlic confit because this is a spontaneous salad and I never seem to have jars full of garlic confit around when I want them. Instead, I go for the more pungent route and paste up a garlic clove to add to the dressing. Of course, if you have garlic confit on hand, feel free to use it when you make this. Or stick to the original, over-the-top spirit of the dish and add both. The blue cheese is strictly optional. If Daniel is supping with me, I leave it out. But if I'm alone, I pile it on and flash back to those crazy, underage dancing days—from the sedentary comfort of my couch.

**Serves 2 as
a light main course,
4 as an appetizer**

4 strips bacon (6 ounces)
1 large garlic clove, finely chopped
1/4 teaspoon plus 1 pinch kosher salt
1 teaspoon red wine vinegar

[CONTINUED]

1 teaspoon Dijon mustard

2 tablespoons extra-virgin olive oil

4 eggs

8 ounces frisée lettuce

2 scallions, thinly sliced

2 ounces blue cheese, crumbled (about ½ cup)

1. In a hot skillet over medium-high heat, fry the bacon until crisp. Transfer to a paper towel–lined plate to drain. Let cool slightly; crumble.

2. Using a mortar and pestle or the back of a knife, mash the garlic with a pinch of salt until it forms a paste. In a small bowl, whisk together the garlic paste, vinegar, mustard, and ¼ teaspoon salt. Slowly whisk in the oil until it is incorporated.

3. Fill a medium pot three-quarters full with water; bring to a simmer. Crack the eggs, one at a time, into a ramekin. Lower the ramekin to the surface of the water and let the egg slide into it. Use a spoon to gently nudge the white closer to the yolk as it simmers. Cook until the white is just set, about 2 minutes for soft poached eggs. Remove each egg with a slotted spoon.

4. In a large bowl, toss together the frisée, crumbled bacon, scallions, and dressing. Divide the salad among individual serving plates. Top each with a poached egg and a sprinkle of crumbled cheese.

What Else?

- If you don't like frisée, you can make this salad with another hearty green. Slivered raw kale works well, as do romaine lettuce and mature crinkly spinach (though not baby spinach, which will wilt too much under the savory load).

- You can leave the bacon out if you're feeling disinclined toward meat.

- Ditto the cheese; leave it out if your Daniel analogue is coming to dinner.

- If you don't feel like going to the trouble of poaching the eggs—which isn't hard but can be daunting if you're not used to it—go ahead and fry them instead. Or soft-boil them and scoop their wobbly guts onto the salad before tossing.

GARLICKY MUSSELS WITH WHITE WINE AND RAMPS

The first time I ate ramps, I had made them myself, testing a recipe in preparation for going on a book tour with Larry Forgione. Larry was the chef of a revolutionary restaurant called An American Place. It opened in the '80s when most fancy restaurants were French, and the idea that all the ingredients used could come from America was startling—an early manifestation of the locavore movement before it was par for the course with chefs.

I worked at his restaurant through college, mostly as a coat-check girl. But Larry knew that I had more food writerly aspirations and agreed to let me accompany him on his book tour as his assistant—back in the era when publishers paid for such things as traveling assistants. Those were the good old, deep-pocketed expense account days; the highlight of the trip was spending the night at the Beverly Hills Hotel, where my room was twice the size of my East Village apartment and about a million times more deluxe. I did a Snoopy dance when I entered the room, and never wanted to leave.

But back to the ramps. I needed to practice making Larry's recipe for goat cheese wrapped in country ham and served with morels and ramps because it was one of the dishes he'd be demo-ing on TV and it was my job to prep all the requisite ingredients.

I'd never so much as seen a ramp before that day, but Larry gave me some to play with, and as I carried home the pungent allium bouquet, I breathed in their lily-like scent.

Back in my kitchen, I peeled and trimmed the ramps like scallions, which they resembled, though the leaves are flatter and thinner, the bulbs more bulbous.

The trick to using them, Larry told me, is to briefly sauté the sliced bulbs as you would garlic, then add the leaves at the end of cooking so they just wilt into the dish. It's still the technique I use whenever I can get ramps, adding them to pastas, sautés, egg dishes, and, in this case, a pot full of briny, winey, absolutely delectable mussels. And like the ramps, I got local mussels at the farmers' market, of which Larry and his apostles certainly would approve.

Serves 2

1 bunch ramps (about 4 ounces), bottoms trimmed
2 tablespoons olive oil
1 small head green garlic or 2 garlic cloves, minced
4 thyme sprigs
Kosher salt or coarse sea salt and freshly ground black pepper
1/2 cup dry white wine
2 pounds mussels, rinsed (see What Else?)
2 tablespoons butter
Crusty bread, for serving

1. Remove the leaves from the ramps and finely chop them; thinly slice the white bulbs.
2. In a large pot over medium-high heat, warm the olive oil. Add the sliced ramp bulbs, garlic, thyme, and a pinch of salt and pepper and sauté until softened, about 2 minutes.
3. Pour in the wine and bring it to a boil. Let simmer until reduced by half, about 4 minutes, then add the mussels and cover the pot. Let the mussels steam, stirring once or twice, until they open, 5 to 10 minutes. Use a slotted spoon to transfer the mussels to bowls. Discard any that have not opened.
4. Add the butter and ramp greens to the pan juices and bring to a boil. Whisk until the butter melts, then taste and correct the seasonings. Pour over the mussels and serve with crusty bread for sopping up the juices.

What Else?

• Wrapped in a damp paper towel, placed in a heavy-duty plastic bag, and stored in your refrigerator's crisper, ramps will keep for weeks. So buy lots when you see them.

[CONTINUED]

- These days, if you are buying mussels at your local fishmonger, chances are they're farmed. This isn't a bad thing. Unlike some other farmed fish with ominous-sounding practices, mussel farming is low impact, and the mussels themselves are very sustainable, not to mention cheap. Another bonus: They've been debearded and thoroughly cleaned before they hit the store, meaning all they need is a quick rinse when you get them home, no shell scraping required.

    Of course, if you've got access to wild mussels, count your blessings. It's true that they will be muddier (or sandier) and likely unshaven, meaning they will need a good scrub and scrape with a paring knife to pull out the byssal threads, also known as beards. But the flavor will be much funkier and more complex than the mild farmed ones. In any case, use what you can get and you won't be sorry.

- When ramps fade out of season, make this with scallions, tender leeks, or spring onions.

A Dish by Another Name

- For Garlicky Clams with White Wine and Ramps, substitute 2 dozen littleneck clams for the mussels. They will take a few extra minutes to cook.

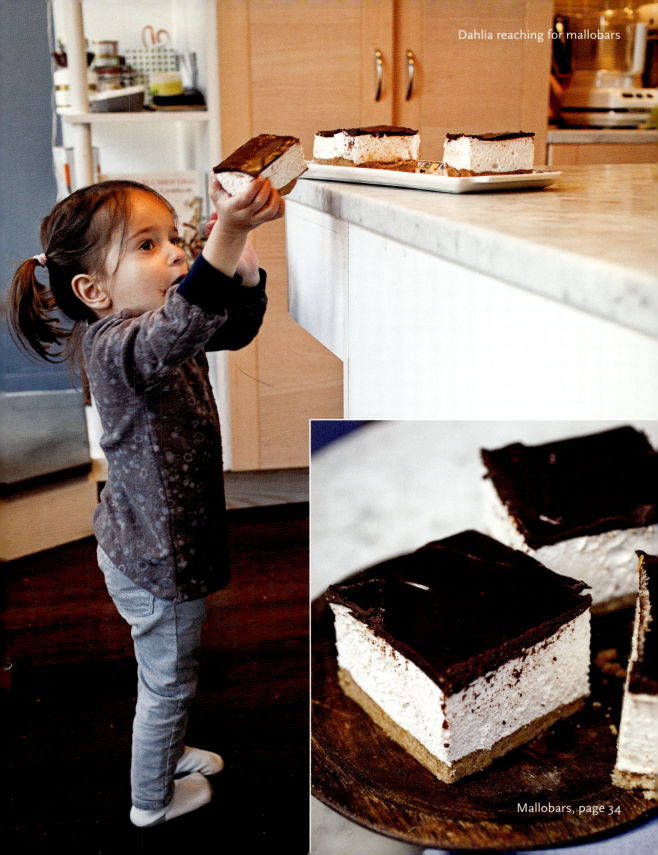

Mallobars, page 34

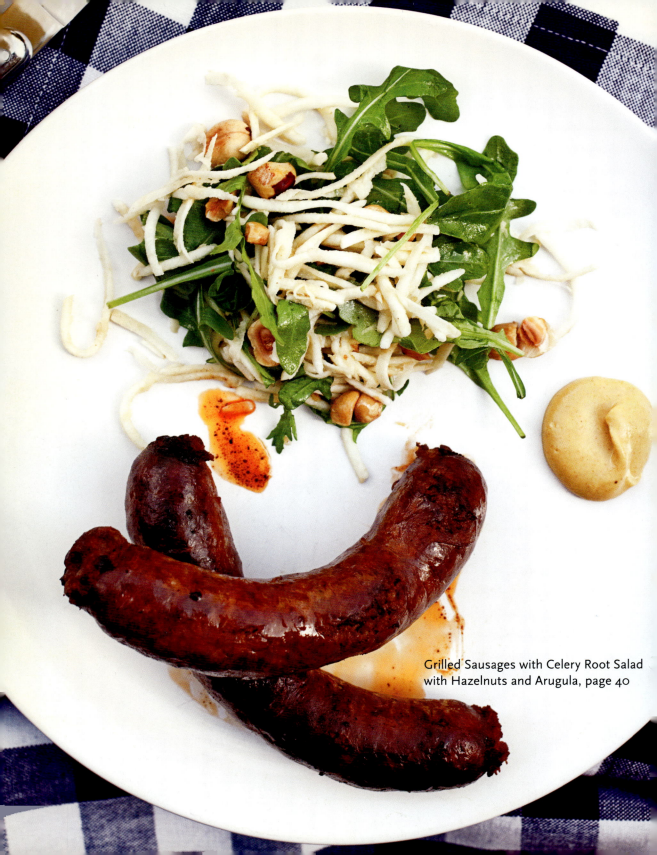

Grilled Sausages with Celery Root Salad with Hazelnuts and Arugula, page 40

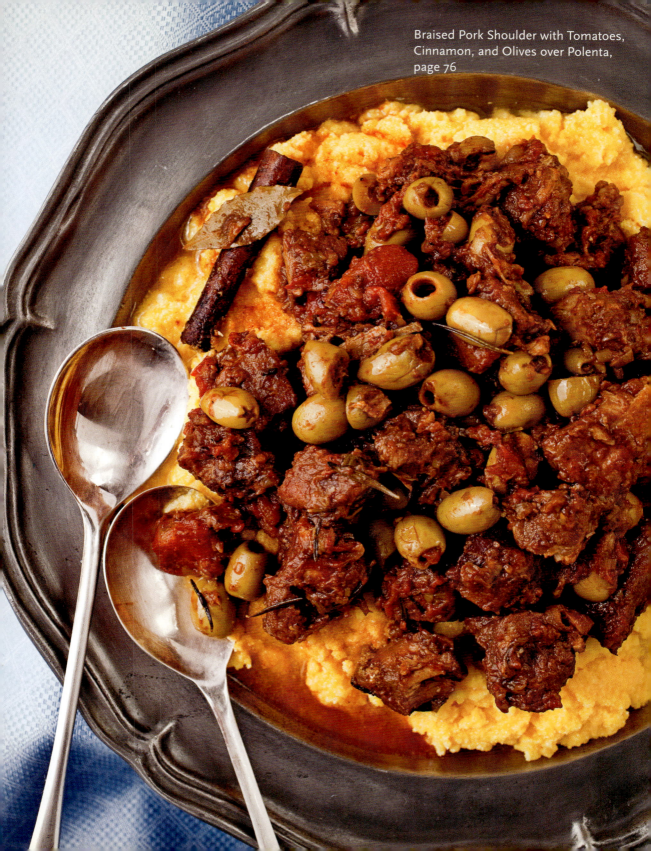

Braised Pork Shoulder with Tomatoes, Cinnamon, and Olives over Polenta, page 76

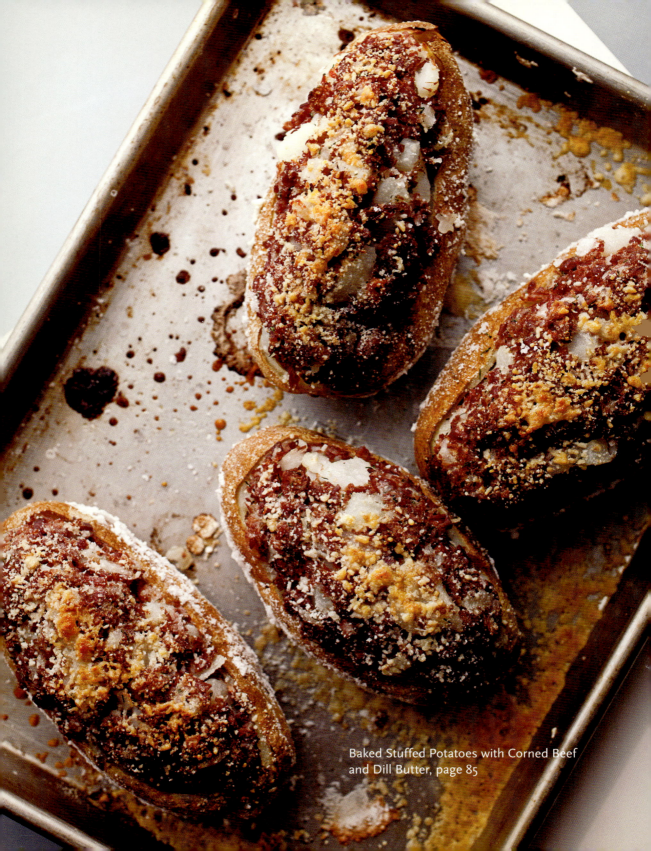

Baked Stuffed Potatoes with Corned Beef and Dill Butter, page 85

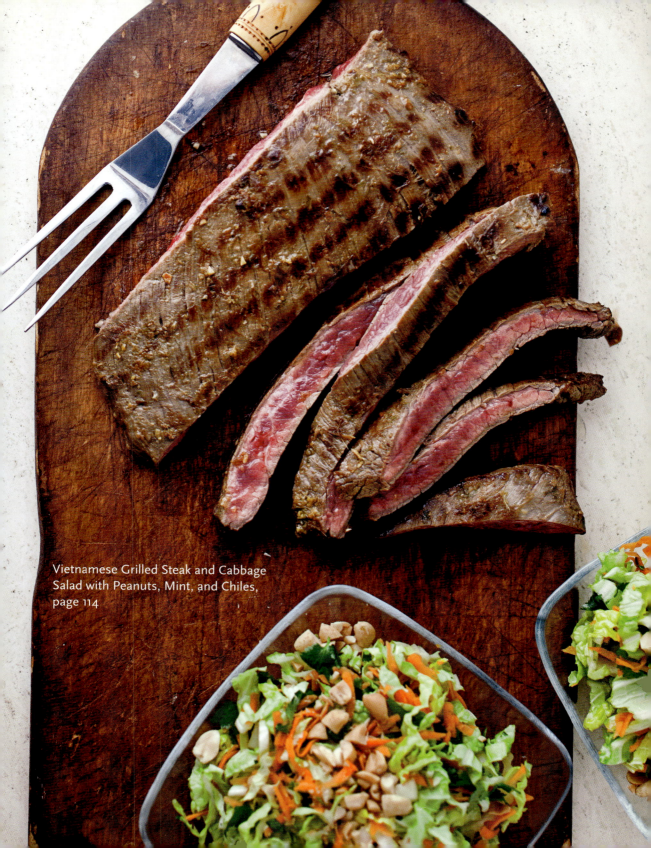

Vietnamese Grilled Steak and Cabbage
Salad with Peanuts, Mint, and Chiles,
page 114

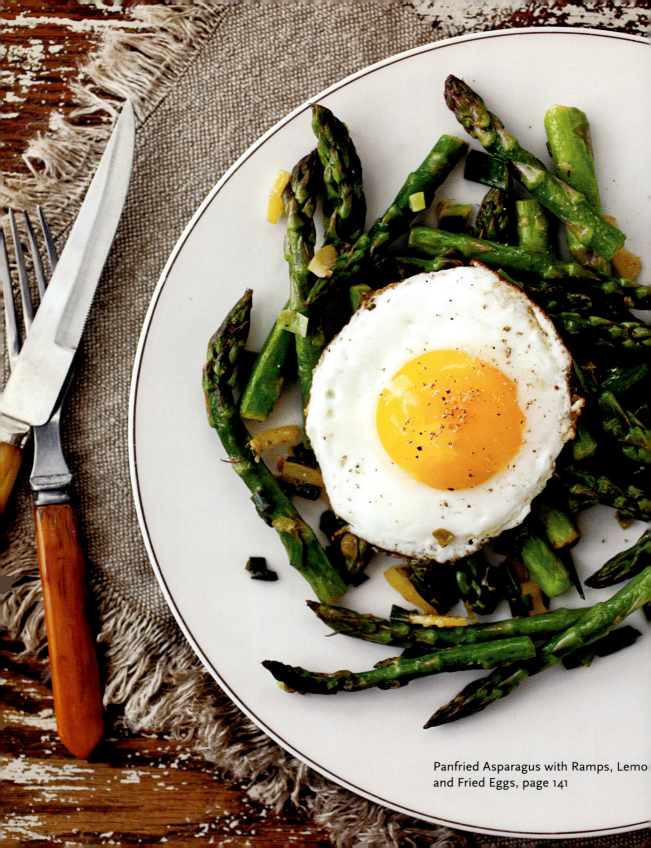

Panfried Asparagus with Ramps, Lemo
and Fried Eggs, page 141

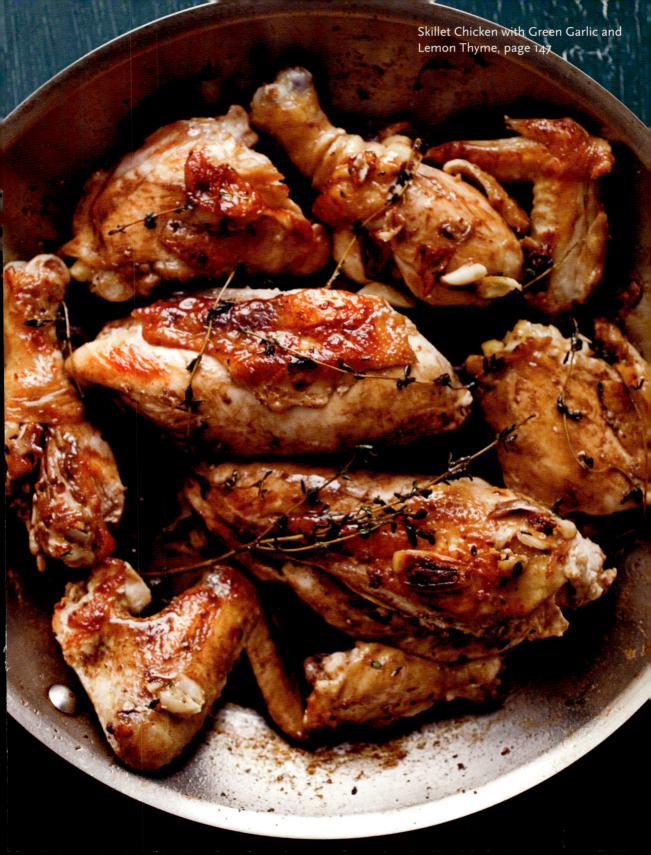

Skillet Chicken with Green Garlic and
Lemon Thyme, page 147

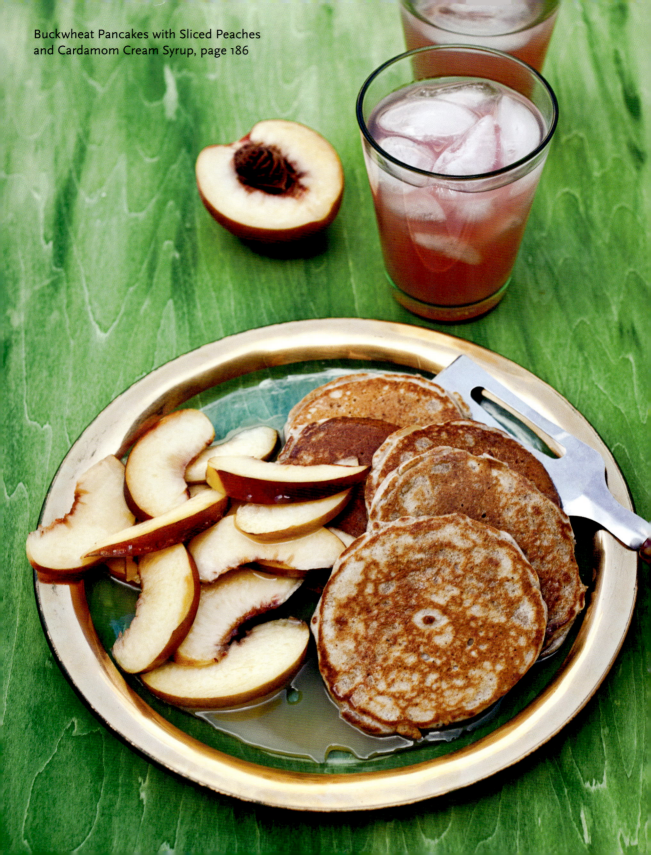

Buckwheat Pancakes with Sliced Peaches
and Cardamom Cream Syrup, page 186

PANFRIED ASPARAGUS WITH RAMPS, LEMON, AND FRIED EGGS

Springtime is all about sharp, raw, biting greens—ramps, chives, nettles—flavors to wake you up after winter's starchy slumber; flavors that say, hey, the snow is melting and here I come, up to the sun. I embrace this. I always buy as many ramps as I can and I find many uses for them. In this recipe, they're sautéed with asparagus, lemon wedges, and eggs. It's one of those odd-sounding but serendipitous combinations, each ingredient bolstering the next—the oniony ramps sweetening the earthy asparagus, which are brightened by the lemon. And the eggs add richness to all. I made this about a dozen times last spring when all the ingredients were in season, and now that they're gone, I'm counting the days until I can make it again. It's that good.

Serves 2 to 4

1 bunch ramps (about 4 ounces), bottoms trimmed

1/4 cup (1/2 stick) unsalted butter

3/4 teaspoon kosher salt, plus additional for seasoning

1/4 teaspoon freshly ground black pepper, plus additional for seasoning

3 thin lemon slices, each round cut into 8 wedges

1 bunch asparagus (about 1/2 pound), trimmed and cut
   into 2-inch pieces

4 large eggs

1. Remove the leaves from the ramps and finely chop them; thinly slice the white bulbs.
2. In a large skillet over medium-high heat, melt 2 tablespoons butter. Sprinkle the skillet with 1/2 teaspoon salt and 1/8 teaspoon pepper. Add the sliced ramp bulbs and lemon wedges and cook, stirring, until slightly softened, about 2 minutes.

[CONTINUED]

3. Add 1 tablespoon butter to the skillet. Stir in the asparagus, chopped ramp leaves, and remaining ¼ teaspoon salt and ⅛ teaspoon pepper. Cover and cook, shaking the pan occasionally, until the asparagus is tender, 4 to 5 minutes. Scrape the mixture onto a plate.

4. Add the remaining 1 tablespoon butter to the skillet. Crack the eggs into the skillet and sprinkle with salt and pepper. Cook the eggs until the edges are set, about 2 minutes. Reduce the heat to medium, cover the pan, and cook until the eggs are completely set, about 1 minute more. Serve the eggs immediately, topped with the warm asparagus mixture.

What Else?

- I've made this using chopped-up preserved lemons instead of the fresh triangles, and it's even better, if you happen to have preserved lemons sitting in your fridge. We always have them in ours; Daniel went through a spate of making his own and we got addicted. You can find them in Middle Eastern stores, and more and more large grocery stores are carrying them. Meyer lemons, preserved or otherwise, work gorgeously here, too.

- When ramp season is done, try using a combination of leeks and garlic as a substitute.

- If you can get your hands on some plump morels, which are often on offer at the farmers' market in spring, wipe them down with a damp cloth, slice them up, and add them to the pan along with the lemon wedges. You might have to add on a few extra minutes of cooking time since the mushrooms will exude a lot of juice and slow things down. Don't use more than a handful, or the mixture might get too wet.

ROASTED ASPARAGUS WITH GINGERED RHUBARB SAUCE

One day a few years ago, my friend Robin called to ask what she should do with all the rhubarb she just carried home from the farmers' market. She happened to call while I was in the middle of deconstructing all that rhubarb *I* had just brought home from the farmers' market, so while I trimmed and chopped, I talked her through it, explaining that because rhubarb takes up so much fridge space, I like to cook it as soon as I get home, and watch a two-pound bag of unwieldy stalks melt into a nice, neat quart of compote.

As I was telling her this, I realized that because of my obsession with guarding my precious little fridge space, I always did the same thing with my rhubarb: Make rhubarb ginger compote.

Not that there is anything wrong with having a steady supply of rhubarb ginger compote to spoon onto yogurt for breakfast. But it was starting to feel like time to branch out, maybe onto the savory side. After all, rhubarb is a vegetable, so why not treat it like one?

Since I love the combination of rhubarb and ginger, I decided to try simmering up a ginger-scented, brown butter rhubarb sauce to spoon over a piece of wild salmon. It was a play on my beloved salmon with brown butter cucumbers recipe (page 168), and I knew the dish would not only look gorgeous—with the pink fish and scarlet sauce—but I was sure the acid in the rhubarb would be a perfect complement to the richness of the fish.

It turns out I was dead wrong. The fish and sauce rebelled against one another, clashing and biting in the most unpleasant way. So Daniel and I scraped the sauce off the fish and ate the salmon naked, which was all well and good because wild salmon doesn't really need anything (other than not overcooking it) to make it taste amazing.

The sauce probably would have just gotten wiped into the trash and I

[CONTINUED]

would have slunk back to my compote-making ways had not a little of it splashed the roasted asparagus that was also sitting on my plate. So I took a bite.

Asparagus and rhubarb is not a flavor combination I ever would have come up with on my own. They're both too big and bossy, I thought, to play well together.

Once again, I was wrong. The two powerful personalities got along beautifully, with the pungent sauce taming the assertive grassiness of the stalks while bringing out their sweetness. It's since become my new favorite rhubarb dish, regardless of my fridge space.

Serves 2 to 4

1 pound thick asparagus, ends snapped
1 tablespoon olive oil
Kosher salt or coarse sea salt and freshly ground black pepper to taste
2 tablespoons butter, or more to taste
1 small head green garlic or 2 garlic cloves, minced
1 tablespoon grated ginger (from a 3/4-inch chunk)
1/4 pound rhubarb, thinly sliced
1 to 2 teaspoons honey, or even more to taste
Chopped chives, for garnish

1. Preheat the oven to 450°F. On a large, rimmed baking pan, toss the asparagus with the oil, salt, and pepper. Spread the stalks out in an even layer and roast until the tips are golden brown, 10 to 15 minutes, depending upon how thick they are.

2. Meanwhile, melt the butter in a large skillet over medium-high heat, and let it cook until it turns deep golden brown and smells nutty, about 5 minutes. Add the garlic, ginger, and a large pinch of salt and pepper and cook until the garlic turns opaque, about a minute. Stir in the rhubarb, cover the pan, and let cook until the rhubarb melts into the sauce, about 5 minutes. Stir in the honey to taste. This will depend upon how sour your rhubarb is; just keep adding honey and salt until it tastes right. Then stop. If the sauce is still too intense, you can whisk in a little more butter to mellow it. It should have a deeply pungent character but should not veer into bitterness.

3. Serve the asparagus covered in rhubarb sauce and showered with chives. Use a lot of chives. Rhubarb sauce isn't pretty.

What Else?

- Last year's rhubarb season came and went far too quickly for me to fully experiment with this sauce. Although the salmon was a bust, I think it has chicken potential, and I could see spooning it on top of broiled or grilled chicken parts. It also might work with shrimp, though given how wrong I was with the salmon, I'd proceed with caution, maybe dipping one small, broiled shrimp into the sauce as a test before slathering the whole lot.

- If you don't feel like making a rhubarb sauce, skip it and serve the roasted asparagus naked or showered in cheese. When Daniel isn't around, I especially love to scatter on some crumbled feta about 3 minutes before the asparagus are ready. This softens and heats the cheese without browning or fully melting it.

- Another amazing thing to do with roasted asparagus: Add mushrooms to the pan. You can use any kind of mushroom, but if you see hen-of-the-woods (also known as maitake), these are ideal since they will cook in the same amount of time as the asparagus if you cut them into 1-inch slices. Simply toss them with more olive oil, add a large pinch of salt, and scatter them on top of the asparagus before roasting. Shiitakes are good, too, and easier to get. Remove the stems and slice the caps in half before oiling them up and tossing with the asparagus.

A Dish by Another Name

- To make Rhubarb Ginger Compote, combine 2 pounds of sliced rhubarb with 2 tablespoons grated ginger and plenty of honey or brown sugar. Add

[CONTINUED]

a few spoonfuls of water or orange juice to the pot and bring everything to a simmer. Simmer, covered, until the rhubarb melts, about 7 minutes. Taste and add more honey or sugar as needed. The tartness of the rhubarb varies. For Dahlia, I cut this sauce with sliced apples, making it milder and less sugar dependent. She eats it about two-thirds of the times I offer it to her—not bad odds for a toddler.

SKILLET CHICKEN WITH GREEN GARLIC AND LEMON THYME

Sautéed chicken is the kind of basic dish that every cook should have a version of in his or her repertoire. It's the essence of easy—the chicken pieces are seasoned with plenty of herbs, then cooked in a skillet in butter and a little wine until the skin turns golden and caramelized and the meat starts to fall off the bone.

You can flavor it with almost any herbs, vegetables, and aromatics that you have around. In spring, I always use green garlic, mostly because in spring I use green garlic for everything. I spend all winter long dreaming of the fresh, tangy flavor of the green-stemmed bulbs, and when the first tiny sprouts appear in the market, I rejoice and use them in pretty much anything I can—except maybe dessert (though I might even go there one day, since my dad has been lobbying for a green garlic sorbet for the past few years).

This said, don't let a lack of green garlic stop you from making this dish. It's excellent with regular garlic, though if yours is old and sprouting, you might want to cut out the green shoot in the center. I don't usually bother, but Daniel always does when he acts as sous-chef. You could also substitute garlic scapes, the jade-colored, loopy shoots of a garlic plant. They don't caramelize in the same way as the bulbs, acting more like a pungent, intense vegetable rather than a true aromatic. Or use a combination of shoots and bulbs, and be prepared to revel in the sweet garlicky flavor of spring.

Serves 4

1 (3½-pound) chicken, cut into 8 pieces
1 tablespoon extra-virgin olive oil
1 teaspoon kosher salt
½ teaspoon freshly ground black pepper
1 bunch fresh thyme (preferably lemon thyme)

[CONTINUED]

1 head green garlic, thickly sliced, or 4 regular garlic cloves,
   peeled and smashed
3/4 cup dry white wine
2–3 tablespoons unsalted butter
Quinoa with Black Pepper, Brown Butter, and Arugula (recipe follows),
   for serving

1. In a large shallow dish, place the chicken, oil, salt, pepper, thyme, and garlic, and mix to coat the chicken. Cover the dish and chill in the refrigerator
   for 2 hours and up to overnight. If you're pressed for time, let the dish
   stand, covered, at room temperature for 30 minutes.

2. In a large skillet over medium heat, place the chicken and seasoning mixture. Cook, without moving the chicken, for 10 minutes. Use a spatula to
   press lightly on the wings to let them get brown. Flip the chicken pieces,
   cover the pan, and continue cooking, without moving, for another 15 to 20
   minutes.

3. Check the breasts by piercing them with a fork to see if they are cooked
   through. If they are, transfer them to a plate and cover with foil to keep
   warm. If not, allow them to cook for another 5 minutes or so, until done.

4. After removing the breasts, use a spoon to take out some of the excess fat.
   Pour in the wine. Simmer, scraping up the brown bits at the bottom of the
   skillet, until the sauce reduces and the remaining chicken parts are cooked
   through, about 5 minutes more. Transfer the chicken to a plate and whisk
   the butter into the pan, whisking until the sauce thickens. Serve with the
   sauce on top of the chicken and don't forget to eat the garlic.

What Else?

- You can use almost the entire green garlic plant—the white bulb and even
  some of the greens—without peeling anything. That's because in their in-
  fant state, green garlic bulbs are as tender as scallions. Once you start to
  see their outer layers of skin toughen and turn papery, then you should
  peel them off. It's a judgment call on the part of the cook.

- This great, basic recipe is adaptable to every season. In summer, add ripe tomatoes and fresh mint or basil to the pan; in autumn, mushrooms and Swiss chard; and in winter, shredded cabbage or winter squash will work wonders to pep up a chilly evening.

- I like this dish with tarragon, too. Substitute about half a bunch for the full bunch of thyme, since tarragon has a stronger flavor.

- If you are using regular thyme, you could mimic the lemony flavor by grating the zest of a lemon into the sauce during the last few minutes of cooking. This adds a nice, bright note. If you are using lemon thyme but absolutely love lemon, you could still do this. The fresh, bright flavor will taste like summer.

- If you'd rather not use the wine, use chicken broth spiked with a few tablespoons of lemon juice for acidity. Dry white vermouth is a good wine substitute if you have an open bottle in your fridge, waiting for the next martini.

- If you aren't planning to make the quinoa, serve a crusty loaf of bread with the chicken to mop up the juices. The bread will also make a cushion upon which to mash the softened, caramelized garlic.

- I also like serving this dish with polenta to absorb all the yummy, buttery pan drippings.

QUINOA WITH BLACK PEPPER, BROWN BUTTER, AND ARUGULA

Before I started cooking more actively with whole grains, I always got amaranth, quinoa, and millet mixed up. I knew that I liked two of them and hated the third. But since I could never remember which was which, I just ignored all three and reached for the couscous when I wanted a quick-cooking, nubby little grain to serve as a side dish.

Many whole grain dishes later, I figured out that it's only the amaranth I don't care for, and that millet and especially quinoa are tasty, nutritious, and relatively fast to cook up. I like them cold, in salads, and warm in pilaf-like side dishes such as this one, which is simple, pretty, adaptable (see What Else?), and very, very good for you, despite the generous drizzle of brown butter. And the arugula adds just the right green bite that makes it taste like spring.

1 cup quinoa

2 tablespoons unsalted butter

2 garlic cloves, minced

4 ounces baby arugula (about 4 cups)

3/4 teaspoon kosher salt

1/2 teaspoon freshly ground black pepper

Serves 2

1. Bring a large pot of salted water to a boil. Add the quinoa and cook until the center is opaque and the husks begin to loosen from the grain, 10 to 12 minutes. Drain well.

2. Melt the butter in a medium skillet over medium heat. Cook until the foam subsides and the butter just begins to turn a nutty brown, about 2 minutes (watch it carefully to see that it doesn't burn). Stir in the garlic and cook 30 seconds. Add the arugula, 1/4 teaspoon salt, and the pepper. Cook, tossing

until the greens are just wilted, about 1 minute. Stir in the quinoa and the remaining ½ teaspoon salt and heat through for 30 seconds; serve.

What Else?

- Swap in cooked millet, whole wheat couscous, or even amaranth (if that's your thing) for the quinoa.

- It's pronounced "KEEN-wah." I'm just saying.

- Baby spinach makes a good stand-in for arugula. Or, if the only green things on hand are herbs, chop up a couple of tablespoons and stir them in. Basil, mint, and cilantro work well.

- This is really good with some grated cheese mixed in, though I pretty much think everything is good with a little cheese mixed in.

- If you want to fancify this, you can add dried cranberries or cherries during the last minute or two of cooking. A garnish of toasted pine nuts or slivered almonds is an elegant touch.

- If you want to use green garlic here, by all means go for it. Use half a large bulb or an entire small one. Or substitute scallions if you'd prefer an oniony flavor. Then use the thinly sliced greens as a garnish.

WHOLE WHEAT BISCUITS WITH SPICY CARDAMOM BUTTER

After writing seven Southern cookbooks with various Southern food experts, including Paula Deen and Sylvia Woods (from Sylvia's in Harlem), I've learned a thing or two about biscuits.

One is that if you're in the company of any good cook from the South, let them make the biscuits. They will probably be better at it than you. It's in their blood, in the way matzo brei is in mine (see page 109).

That said, there are some tips to making truly light and flaky biscuits, the kind that break apart into buttery layers when you greedily pull the top off before smearing on even more butter (or gravy if you're from the South).

The first is to use a light touch, making sure not to overmix the dough. You want to keep the butter in pieces as you would when making pie dough. Those little chunks melt in the oven, producing steam that creates the characteristic flakes. Another important biscuit rule is to go through whatever hoops necessary to serve them warm from the oven, slathered with even more butter. Cold biscuits, while good, are never extraordinary (though toasted they are pretty darn tasty; see What Else?).

I know my Southern friends will likely look askance at my whole wheat version. But I love the rich, roasty flavor of the whole wheat flour here, which gives the biscuits a deep complexity. They are also wonderfully light, even given their bran content. The cardamom butter, slightly sweet and very fragrant, is a nice match but purely optional. And if you've got homemade jam, such as the Rhubarb, Strawberry, and Lemon Marmalade on page 158, it will be most welcome here, with or without the cardamom butter.

1 cup all-purpose flour, plus additional for the table

2/3 cup whole wheat flour

1 1/2 tablespoons baking powder

1/4 teaspoon kosher salt

6 tablespoons (3/4 stick) cold unsalted butter, cut into cubes

2/3 cup whole milk

1 tablespoon honey

1 tablespoon unsalted butter, melted

Rhubarb, Strawberry, and Lemon Marmalade (page 158)
    or other jam (optional)

FOR THE SPICY CARDAMOM BUTTER

1 stick (8 tablespoons) butter, softened

1 1/2 tablespoons honey

1/2 teaspoon ground cardamom, pinch more to taste if it needs it

1/8 teaspoon kosher salt

1/8 teaspoon cayenne

1. Preheat the oven to 400°F. Line a rimmed baking sheet with parchment paper.

2. Place the flours, baking powder, and salt in the bowl of a food processor and pulse to combine.

3. Add the cold butter and pulse until the mixture resembles coarse meal. Pour in the milk, drizzle in the honey, and continue pulsing until the dough starts to come together, scraping down the sides of the bowl if necessary.

4. Turn the dough onto a lightly floured surface and gently pat it together. Use a floured biscuit cutter (2 to 3 inches) to cut out the biscuits. Transfer the biscuits to the prepared baking sheet, brush with the melted butter, and bake until golden brown, 15 to 18 minutes. Transfer the pan to a wire rack to cool for a few minutes (but not much longer) before serving.

5. While the biscuits are baking, prepare the cardamom butter by beating all the ingredients together with an electric mixer or in a food processor. Add more honey, salt, or spice to taste. Spread on the warm biscuits.

What Else?

- If you don't want to bother with the cardamom butter—or if it sounds too weird for you—just skip it and slather in plenty of regular butter instead. Or make cinnamon butter, substituting ground cinnamon for the cardamom. It will have a spicy-sweet flavor that's especially nice around the holidays.

- Sometimes if I'm feeling too lazy to melt more butter for brushing the tops of the biscuits before baking them, I'll just brush on some cream or milk. It gets them nearly as brown and is easier.

- Make these into strawberry sandwiches by splitting the biscuits, spreading them with cardamom butter, and stuffing them with sliced sugared strawberries. They make a terrific breakfast and a satisfying, almost shortcake-like midafternoon snack.

- These biscuits freeze really well. Wrap them in a layer of plastic wrap, then in foil. When ready to reheat, let them thaw at room temperature for an hour or so, then split them in half and run them under the broiler until toasted. Serve with plenty of butter. They aren't as light as they are when fresh, but whenever I have leftovers, this is what I do.

RHUBARB CURD SHORTBREAD TART WITH FRESH STRAWBERRIES

For years, all I ever did when combining strawberries and rhubarb was make pie. I don't even particularly love strawberry rhubarb pie. I never order it at restaurants and don't crave it when the season is done. It's a nice pie, though not in the sour cherry–apple crumb–coconut cream league. But I made it nonetheless, partly out of a desire to cleave to tradition and partly out of a rare instance of culinary complacency.

But last spring, as I gathered my quarts of nice, tiny strawberries and bags of leggy rhubarb from the farmers' market, I rebelled. The time had come to do something different. And besides, the wee strawberries I was able to snag were so deeply sweet and aromatic, it seemed a shame to cook them at all. They needed to be enthroned on the shortbread cookie pastry of a fresh fruit tart, not melted and hidden beneath a piecrust.

But I didn't want to forgo my beloved strawberry rhubarb combination entirely, and I had several options for incorporating the rhubarb into the tart. I could have made jam and used it for the bottom. I could have candied bits of the stalks and strewn them on top. But in the end, I decided to make rhubarb curd. Curd is one of those creamy, buttery custards that Daniel can actually eat since there is no cream or milk in it, and I love a creamy texture with the bright acidity of raw fruit.

I made the tart, adding a touch of cardamom and orange zest to my favorite shortbread crust recipe to give it more oomph. Then I spread the pale pink rhubarb curd on top, covering it with just enough of the tiny berries to seem lush and inviting, but still leaving some bare spots so the pretty curd would peek through.

It was certainly more beautiful than my usual strawberry rhubarb pie, and much more thrilling to eat, with the hint of spice and crunch of the

[CONTINUED]

cookie crust complementing the juicy berries and the creamy, tangy curd. And unlike the pie, six months after the last crumb was devoured and rhubarb season has come and gone, I'm craving this tart as I type. A new spring tradition has just been born.

Makes 1 (9-inch) tart
Serves 6 to 8

FOR THE SHORTBREAD TART CRUST

1 1/2 cups all-purpose flour

1/4 cup confectioners' sugar, plus additional for serving

1 tablespoon freshly grated orange zest

1/2 teaspoon kosher salt

1/4 teaspoon ground cardamom

12 tablespoons unsalted butter, chilled and cut into cubes

FOR THE RHUBARB CURD

10 ounces rhubarb, trimmed and cut into 1-inch pieces (about 3 cups)

1/2 cup plus 1 tablespoon sugar

4 egg yolks

2 eggs

1/4 teaspoon kosher salt

6 tablespoons unsalted butter, chopped into pieces

About 2 cups strawberries, hulled and halved, or thickly sliced if large

1. To make the crust, place the flour, confectioners' sugar, orange zest, salt, and cardamom in the bowl of a food processor with the blade attachment and pulse to combine. Add the butter and run the motor just until a crumbly dough forms.

2. Scrape the dough into a 9-inch tart pan. Use your fingers to press the dough into and up the sides of the pan. Use a spatula to smooth the bottom, then chill in the refrigerator for 30 minutes.

3. Preheat the oven to 325°F. Line the tart dough with a sheet of foil and fill with pie weights. Bake until light golden brown, 35 to 40 minutes.

4. While the crust is baking, prepare the curd. Puree the rhubarb in a food processor until smooth, about 2 to 3 minutes (add a few teaspoons of

water if necessary to help the rhubarb move, though try to keep this to a minimum so it doesn't dilute the juice). Pour into a bowl lined with cheesecloth. Tighten the cheesecloth and squeeze out the juice with your hands, discarding the pulp. You should get about 2/3 cup of juice.

5. In a double boiler or a stainless steel medium bowl set on top of a medium heavy-bottomed pot with 2 inches of simmering water, combine the rhubarb juice, sugar, egg yolks, eggs, and salt. Stir constantly, with a whisk, making sure to scrape the bottom and sides, while the liquid thickens and coats the back of a wooden spoon, about 18 to 20 minutes. Remove from heat and whisk in butter until dissolved.

6. Strain the curd through a fine-mesh sieve.

7. When the crust is ready, take it out of the oven, remove the foil and pie weights, and lower the oven temperature to 300°F. Spread the rhubarb curd into the tart shell and smooth with a spatula. Bake for another 10 minutes, until the curd is just set. Transfer the tart to a wire rack to cool completely, at least 1 hour.

8. Just before serving, scatter the strawberries over the tart and sprinkle with confectioners' sugar. Serve at once.

What Else?

• Rhubarb and strawberries may be classic, but raspberries make a nice topper here, too, if you can get them.

• The rhubarb curd is delicious on its own, as a topping for a big bowl of sugared berries, or on top of pound cake or biscuits.

• Believe me, I hate straining, and would not inflict it upon you if the texture weren't really so much lovelier without the stringy rhubarb bits. However, if you really don't want to strain and you don't mind the texture, then don't do it. It's your tart, after all, and as long as you are happy, your guests will be, too (or at least they won't say anything to your face . . .).

RHUBARB, STRAWBERRY, AND LEMON MARMALADE

This is what I do with springtime strawberries that aren't pretty enough to sit on top of a tart. I make them into jam, adding rhubarb and a little lemon to brighten their intense sweetness.

I got the basic technique for this jam from the French jam-making guru Christine Ferber. She makes the most incredible jams I've ever tasted, and when she came out with a cookbook a few years ago, I adopted it as my pre-serving bible.

At first, however, I was skeptical about the need to macerate the fruit overnight in sugar. Can't one just boil it longer and not bother? But having made jams both ways, I can tell you that macerating really does make a huge difference in texture. It allows the fruit to candy and absorb some of the sugar before it hits the heat, which helps it maintain its texture rather than falling apart to mush.

This recipe gives you a translucent, lemony jelly packed with candied chunks of strawberry and rhubarb. It's excellent on toast or biscuits (page 152), though I often find myself eating it off the spoon in winter when I want a sugary treat that reminds me of the sweetness of spring.

1¼ pounds rhubarb, washed, trimmed, and diced
    (about 4½ cups)
1½ pounds strawberries, washed, trimmed, and diced
    (about 6 cups)
4½ cups sugar
Freshly grated zest of 1 lemon
Freshly squeezed juice of ½ lemon

4 to 6 sterilized jam jars, depending upon size
    (see What Else?)

Makes about 6 cups

1. In a large bowl, place the rhubarb, strawberries, sugar, lemon zest, and lemon juice. Cover and let sit, stirring occasionally, 6 to 8 hours or overnight.

2. Put a small plate or saucer in the freezer. Place a sieve over a large saucepan and pour the fruit mixture into the sieve, reserving the fruit for later. Affix a candy thermometer to the side of the saucepan and place over medium-high heat. Bring the mixture to a boil and allow to simmer until the temperature reads 230°F, 15 to 20 minutes.

3. Add the reserved fruit and bring the mixture back to a boil, stirring occasionally. Simmer for 5 to 10 minutes. Check to see if the jam will set by placing a small spoonful on the chilled saucer. Push the edge of the jam puddle inward with your finger; if the puddle wrinkles then the jam is done.

4. Ladle the hot jam into the jam jars, leaving 1/2 inch of headspace, and seal tightly. If you want to can the jars, process in a canner according to the manufacturer's directions. Or, for shorter storage, turn the sealed jars upside down and allow them to cool to room temperature (see What Else?). The jar tops should be sealed and look concave. Properly sealed jars will keep in the refrigerator for at least several months or in the pantry for at least several weeks. If some jars don't seal, store them in the fridge and use them up first.

What Else?

- I never can my jams with a pressure canner, preferring to make small batches of jam and use them up quickly. This is my method. (Please note that this does not comply with the USDA recommendations for safe canning.) If you have a dishwasher, wash the jars and lids (use the sterilize setting if you've got one) and take them out while they're still hot. Or, you can boil the jars and the lids for 10 minutes. Set them upside down on a clean dishtowel to dry. Then ladle the hot jam into the hot jars, leaving 1/2 inch of headspace, and screw on the lids while everything is still steaming hot. Turn them upside down and allow a vacuum seal to occur. You will know that the jars are sealed in a vacuum if the tops of the jars look concave. This will preserve them for weeks and probably months. If you see mold, toss the jam. Note that botulism isn't an issue with jam-making because of the high acid and sugar content, so you don't need to worry about that. But moldy jam isn't tasty.

- If you don't feel like dealing with any of this, just store the jam in the fridge and use it up in the next few months. Or pop it into the freezer for longer storage.

JUNE

PAN-ROASTED RADISH AND ANCHOVY CROSTINI

The first time I ate a roasted radish at a friend's house for dinner, I thought it was a baby turnip—a sweet, tender, caramelized turnip with a faint mustard edge to give it verve.

I gobbled up an entire plateful before realizing that, in fact, I was eating radishes. The pink skins and oblong shape finally clued me in.

It's probably a good thing I didn't know what I was nibbling before I was hooked. Because before I discovered otherwise, cooked radishes did not sound at all appealing. In my mind, radishes were supposed to be crunchy, taut, and a little bitter, a cleansing vegetable to cut the fat of rich foods.

These sweet little orbs were none of those things. But they were completely beguiling in their own right.

Now, come June when radishes are available at the farmers' market in ruby profusion, cooking them has become an integral part of my radish repertoire. Usually I pan-roast them, which is faster than oven roasting and adds more color, too. They are so flavorful on their own that they don't need more than a slick of olive oil and a sprinkle of salt to bring them to life.

But if you are one for flavorful excess, and I most certainly am, layering them onto a crisp crostini and adding a pungent, buttery anchovy sauce will probably make you smile—in between bites, that is.

Serves 4 to 6

1 bunch radishes

1/4 cup plus 1 1/2 tablespoons extra-virgin olive oil

1/2 teaspoon kosher salt

1/4 teaspoon freshly ground black pepper

4 tablespoons (1/2 stick) unsalted butter

8 anchovy fillets, finely chopped

4 fat garlic cloves, finely chopped

Pinch red pepper flakes
Fresh lemon juice to taste
8 ($\frac{1}{2}$-inch-thick) slices crusty bread, toasted
4 teaspoons chopped fresh parsley

1. Remove the leaves and stems from the radishes; trim the tails. Cut the large radishes lengthwise into sixths and the smaller radishes lengthwise into quarters.

2. Heat a large skillet over medium-high heat until very hot. Add 1½ tablespoons oil. Add the radishes in a single layer (do not crowd the skillet); season with the salt and pepper. Cook the radishes, without moving, until lightly colored on the undersides, about 3 minutes. Shake the pan and continue cooking until fork-tender, about 3 minutes.

3. In a small skillet or saucepan over medium heat, melt the butter. Stir in the remaining ¼ cup oil, anchovies, garlic, and red pepper flakes. Reduce the heat to low and gently simmer until warm, about 4 minutes. Stir in the lemon juice to taste.

4. Brush each slice of toast with the warm anchovy sauce and top with several radish wedges. Spoon additional sauce on top. Sprinkle each toast with parsley and serve.

What Else?

- Using all olive oil in the sauce works just as well as the butter–olive oil combination I suggest here, so feel free to substitute as you see fit.

- The anchovy sauce is absolutely amazing on nearly everything, so even if you hate radishes, try making the sauce at least once. It's so robust and garlicky that you can spoon it on toasted bread, call it anchovy crostini, and everyone you serve it to will be delighted. Just don't tell them radishes were supposed to be there and they will never know.

[CONTINUED]

- I suppose you could make this recipe without the anchovies if you really hate them. In which case, I would top the crostini with some good Parmigiano-Reggiano, shaved into curls, to give the dish an umami pop.

- If you skip the bread, this makes a really unusual side dish. Just toss the radishes into the anchovy sauce and serve. It's excellent with roast chicken and other birds.

PASTA WITH GARLIC SCAPES PESTO, SUGAR SNAP PEAS, AND RICOTTA

One day I got a call from Adam Roberts, a home cook and blogger otherwise known as the Amateur Gourmet. He'd just scored a cookbook deal and was wondering if I wanted to be part of it, essentially giving him a cooking lesson that he could pass onto his readers and create an original recipe from.

I was flattered, but a little taken aback. I'm not a teacher, so I wasn't sure what kind of useful information I could impart. But he said all I'd have to do was shop with him and his photographer at the farmers' market, where I had to go anyway, and then come home and cook a meal.

Considering I pretty much did this several times a week anyway, it seemed like something I could handle. We met on a gorgeous late spring morning at Union Square and wandered from stand to stand, picking up emerald sugar snap peas, twisty jade garlic scapes, bunches of herbs, handmade eggy pasta, and fresh sheep's milk ricotta. I had no idea what I'd do with it all when we got home, but was prepared to wing it, just as I always do.

Of course, while we were on the subway chitchatting about mucilaginous arugula and other foodie preoccupations, I was simultaneously hatching a plan about what to cook. My first thought was to sauté the scapes and peas with prosciutto, then toss them with the pasta, garnishing with the ricotta. But by the time the train pulled into our stop, I had decided to make pesto out of the garlic scapes and cilantro, and to use the sugar snap peas and ricotta for a simple crostini, garnished with good olive oil and crunchy salt.

That was the first dish we made as soon as we walked in the door, and although we ate every bite, I wasn't perfectly satisfied. Despite their anchor of cheese, the peas kept falling off the crostini and onto the nice clean floor I'd just mopped to impress my camera-wielding visitors. I needed to redeem myself.

[CONTINUED]

Since we had some peas and ricotta left, I decided to throw them into the pasta pesto, and it was a good move, the creamy cheese softening the pungency of the garlic scapes and intense grassiness of the uber-fresh cilantro. It was so delectable that no one noticed that I forgot all about the prosciutto.

Best of all, Dahlia loved the dish, sticking her little fingers into the serving bowl and grabbing fistfuls to stuff in her mouth while I was too busy trying to play both model and food stylist to stop her.

It was an outside-the-quotidian, very fun day in my house. I don't know if Adam learned anything, but we all ate exceedingly well.

1/4 cup pine nuts

Serves 4

3/4 cup cilantro or basil leaves

1/2 cup thinly sliced garlic scapes

1/4 cup good Parmesan cheese, preferably Parmigiano-Reggiano, more to taste

1/2 teaspoon kosher or coarse sea salt, more to taste

1/2 cup extra-virgin olive oil

1 pound cavatelli or other pasta that makes you happy

1 tablespoon butter

1/4 pound sugar snap peas, trimmed and sliced 1/4 inch thick

Freshly ground black pepper

Fresh ricotta, for serving

1. Over medium heat, toast the pine nuts in a small, dry skillet until they start to smell nutty and turn golden, about 3 minutes. Pour the nuts onto a plate to cool.

2. In a food processor or blender, combine the cilantro or basil, garlic scapes, cheese, and salt, and process until the mixture is well combined and the herbs are finely chopped. Add the nuts and oil and process until smooth, scraping down the sides of the bowl occasionally. Taste and add more salt if needed.

3. Bring a large pot of water to a boil and add enough salt to make it taste like the sea (or just very salty if you don't go around sipping the sea). Add the pasta and cook until al dente (subtract a minute or two from the cooking time on the package).

4. While the pasta is cooking, melt the butter in a skillet and add the peas and a pinch of salt. Sauté until they are crisp-tender, about 3 minutes.

5. Drain the pasta and toss with just enough of the pesto to coat it. Season with salt if needed. Top with the peas, sprinkle with more Parmesan cheese and plenty of black pepper, and dollop spoonfuls of fresh ricotta on top.

What Else?

- If you'd rather use shell peas instead of sugar snaps, you will need about a pound. Shell them and throw them in the skillet as you would the sugar snaps.

- I recently learned from my friends over at Franny's restaurant in Brooklyn that a good rule of thumb for salting pasta water is to add about a third of a cup to your average pot of boiling water. That's a lot more than most of us use, but the salty water seasons the pasta so that you don't need to add more salt later. I can attest that this method works very well, though I don't measure so much as eyeball it.

- This is really tasty with some slivered prosciutto tossed in with the peas before they're added to the pasta. Stir in the prosciutto after you've turned off the burner. The residual heat in the pan will be enough to warm it up.

- I make a cheese-free version of the pesto for Daniel by using a little extra salt and adding some lemon zest for complexity. It's nearly as good as the Parmesan version. Sometimes I'll serve Daniel the cheeseless pesto, and then shower my plate with Parmesan before devouring. But if I don't think of it, I honestly don't miss it. The ricotta, however, is another story entirely. I love the stuff, and will dollop it with abandon on anything that stands still long enough to accept the blob. So if I've got it in the fridge, it's going on the pasta, on my portion at least.

SEARED WILD SALMON WITH BROWN BUTTER CUCUMBERS

My year-round visits to the farmers' market has made me in tune with what the cold snap means for the tomatoes or what havoc an early snowfall can have on beans. I know not to look for new potatoes in October or pumpkins in May.

But there is a limit to this knowledge, and it ends at the border of the vegetable kingdom. The minute I step into meat and fish land, I assume that all seasonality has been bred out of the offerings. We no longer have to necessarily butcher pigs in the winter and eat baby lamb in the spring. It's available to us all year long, thanks to modern animal husbandry and subzero freezers.

There are, however, a few exceptions when it comes to protein, and one of them is wild salmon. The best, richest, most tender salmon is summer-caught salmon, before the fish begin their aquatic adventures to spawning ground. Spawning is a vigorous endeavor, and to prepare, they put on a lot of nice, tasty fat, readying themselves for their long swim through cold rushing waters. This makes summer the best time to catch them, and naturally to eat them, too.

This said, you can buy excellent quality frozen wild salmon most of the year, and I do. But when fresh wild salmon is in season, I go out of my way to dig in and I suggest you do the same. Trust me, if you've only ever eaten lackluster farmed salmon, when you get your paws on some fresh, wild-caught stuff, you might never go back.

There are about a zillion ways to cook salmon, and most of them are fine. If I've scored some really good fish, though, I say, the simpler the better, so you can really taste what all the fuss is about.

This recipe is a prime example of a simple preparation. The fish is seasoned minimally with salt and pepper before being seared in brown butter. I could easily end the recipe here and you'd all be very happy (or at least I would be). But swirling in some cucumber cubes, minced garlic, and herbs lifts the dish into the realm of the sublime. The cucumber heats up gently, releasing plenty of juice but staying crisp enough for a textural contrast to the satiny fish. It's such a felicitous combination that it even makes farmed salmon taste extraordinary. And that's really saying something.

Serves 2

2 thick wild salmon fillets (6 to 8 ounces each)
Kosher salt and freshly ground black pepper to taste
2 tablespoons unsalted butter
2 Kirby cucumbers, peeled and diced into 1/4-inch cubes
2 garlic cloves, finely chopped
2 tablespoons chopped fresh basil or mint
Lime wedges, for serving

1. Season the salmon with salt and pepper. In a large skillet over medium-high heat, melt the butter. Cook until the foam subsides and the butter turns deep gold in color, about 2 minutes (watch it carefully to see that it does not burn).
2. Add the salmon to the pan, skin-side up. Cook, without turning, for 2 minutes. Add the cucumbers and a pinch of salt to the pan around the salmon; stir to coat it with the butter. Continue to cook, stirring the cucumbers, until the underside of the fish turns dark golden, about 3 minutes longer. Flip the fish (push the cucumbers to one side of the pan so that the fish can make contact with the pan). Add the garlic to the cucumbers and stir. Cook the fish until done to taste, 2 to 4 minutes longer.
3. Stir the basil or mint into the cucumbers in the pan. Taste and adjust the seasonings, if necessary. Spoon the cucumbers and butter sauce over the fish and serve with lime wedges, encouraging people to squeeze them. This needs a tiny bit of acid to bring out all the flavors.

What Else?

- Boiled soba noodles, dressed with sesame oil and salt, are a great accompaniment here. Rice is nice, too.

[CONTINUED]

- This basic technique will work with almost any kind of fish. Arctic char is another pretty, pale pink possibility (if you choose your fish by color). Just make sure to ask for a thick, center-cut piece. The thinner end pieces tend to overcook. Healthful, sustainable mackerel is good here, too, though it will cook more quickly than the salmon, so watch it carefully. In that case, add a good squeeze of lime juice at the end, since mackerel's meaty-tasting flesh always needs a boost of acidity. Halibut will also work but needs extra careful cooking so it doesn't dry out. Make sure to turn the heat down to low and watch this vulnerable morsel closely (it's done when it's opaque but before it flakes).

- Zucchini makes a summery cucumber alternative. Ditto summer squash. You don't need to peel them, which is nice, and if you use one of each (choose very small specimens), you'll be rewarded with an especially colorful presentation with that gorgeous salmon-hued salmon.

- If you don't have basil or mint, substitute thyme or rosemary branches, adding them to the skillet along with the butter as it's melting. They will perfume the whole pan. Just make sure to remove them before serving the fish.

CRUSHED NEW POTATOES AND PEA SALAD WITH MUSTARD SEED DRESSING

I'd been cooking with and eating new potatoes for years before I finally learned that in fact I had not. Those cute little red potatoes I'd always called "new red potatoes"? Turns out they are not necessarily new at all.

My education came—where else?—at the farmers' market, when Franca Tantillo at Berried Treasures Farm, my favorite strawberry grower at the Union Square Market, proudly showed off a basket of her newly dug potatoes. Upon first inspection, I wasn't excited. They looked like every other potato I'd ever seen, and I was about to walk away without buying any.

"You're missing out. Have you ever had *real* new potatoes?" she asked in a tone that conveyed "obviously not."

She went on to explain that potatoes, like garlic and onions, are such good storing vegetables that they will last the whole winter through. There isn't a season without them at the farmers' market, where they fill the bins week in and week out. And it's because they are so ubiquitous, she said, that they get taken for granted. No one makes a tomato-like fuss when the freshly dug ones hit the farm stands along with the peas in early summer.

So I brought home a bagful and boiled them up for dinner.

And do you know what? New potatoes, with their gossamer-thin skins and moist, almost nutty-tasting flesh, really are different—and better—than old potatoes. They have a rich, buttery flavor that doesn't need a lot of fat to bring it out. I have no problem slathering older potatoes with buckets of butter and/or olive oil, but that would overwhelm these youngsters, which need just a touch of butter and salt to make a memorable side dish all by themselves.

But if you want something with a little more pizzazz, try this savory salad. It's got a little bit of a lot of different elements, and they all work together to

[CONTINUED]

enhance the gentle earthy character of the actually new potatoes, with peas adding a sweet crispness, yogurt lending tanginess, and Dijon mustard and mustard seeds spicing everything up with their warm bite. If you've only got old potatoes to cook with, make this anyway. Then follow Ms. Tantillo's advice and watch for new potatoes when they next come into season. And spread the word; they deserve a bit of fuss.

Serves 4

1 pound new potatoes

3/4 cup fresh shelled peas

3/4 teaspoon black or brown mustard seeds (see What Else?)

3 tablespoons plain yogurt (optional)

2 teaspoons Dijon mustard

2 tablespoons finely chopped shallot

1/2 teaspoon kosher salt

1/4 teaspoon freshly ground black pepper

1 to 3 tablespoons extra-virgin olive oil to taste

2 tablespoons chopped fresh mint or chives

1. Place the potatoes in a large pot of salted water. Bring to a boil and cook until almost tender, about 20 minutes. Drop in the peas and cook until they are tender, 3 to 5 minutes. Drain well.
2. Meanwhile, make the vinaigrette: In a small, dry skillet, toast the mustard seeds until they just begin to pop, about 1 minute. Transfer to a small bowl. Whisk in the yogurt, mustard, shallot, salt, and pepper. Place the warm potatoes and peas in a large bowl and gently crush the potatoes (they should remain almost whole). Add the dressing and olive oil and toss to combine. Fold in the mint or chives. Taste and adjust the seasoning, if necessary. Serve warm.

What Else?

*   Old potatoes will work well here; just choose thin-skinned boiling potatoes in place of thick-skinned bakers. Yukon Gold, which split the difference, are perfectly fine; russets, not so much.

- If you don't have black or brown mustard seeds, leave them out and just add a little more Dijon mustard.

- If you want to leave out the yogurt, add a little more olive oil to keep things moist.

- I love mint with peas, but tarragon is a less obvious and equally tasty choice. Use 1 tablespoon since it's a lot more potent than mint.

- Sometimes I make this with thinly sliced sugar snap peas in place of the shell peas. You'll need about 1/4 pound.

- I've also made this with frozen peas, and they can be sweeter than mediocre fresh peas. Bear in mind, though, that frozen peas will only need about a minute of cooking time, so add them later than you would fresh peas.

CLAMS WITH PEAS, PEA SHOOTS, AND ISRAELI COUSCOUS

When I was growing up, clams were a summer thing, a fried-bellies-at-a-beach-shack thing or throw-them-on-the-grill thing—with the one major exception of chowder, which we ate in winter. But for the most part, clams were part in parcel with fresh sweet corn and sand between your toes.

What we never had in any season was pasta with clam sauce. We didn't cook it, nor did we order it at Tommasso's, our favorite Brooklyn old-school Italian restaurant. It barely registered as an option at all, until the day I finally tried it when I was in college and immediately fell for its garlicky, saline, buttery yumminess. After that, it became my go-to order at any Italian restaurant (white sauce, please).

I didn't start making it myself until a few years ago, when I realized that, given the state of the ocean's ecosystem, clams were one of the few sea creatures I could savor without guilt. Since I loved it anyway, it seemed like a good time to learn how to make pasta with clam sauce a part of my repertoire.

I've made it countless times since then, varying it as I am wont to do, but always respecting the elements that made me fall in love with the flavors in the first place, that heady combination of clams, garlic, and wine.

This is the dish's springtime incarnation. Peas, pea shoots, and green garlic make it especially bright and sweet tasting, while mint adds freshness. I use Israeli couscous here in place of more traditional pasta because I love the way the little pearls feel sliding around in my mouth, swabbed with the tasty sauce. And their round shape reminds me of bubbles, which seems appropriate, given the clams' watery origins.

When I served this dish to my family, I wasn't surprised that Dahlia wouldn't touch the clams (though I had held out a modicum of hope since she loves the salty flavor of salmon roe; but then again, those neon red salmon eggs are prettier than gray clams). However, I was sure that I'd get her to eat some of the Israeli couscous. I even tried renaming them pasta bubbles. But alas, she pushed my hand away with a polite yet emphatic "No, thank you, Mommy," and I had to retreat. I can't honestly say that I minded all that much. In this case, it meant more for me.

Serves 2

2 dozen littleneck clams, scrubbed
3 tablespoons unsalted butter
1/4 cup finely chopped shallots (about 2 small)
1 small head green garlic or 2 fat regular garlic cloves, finely chopped
Pinch red pepper flakes
1/3 cup white wine
2/3 cup fresh peas
1 cup pea shoots
1/4 cup chopped fresh mint
Cooked Israeli couscous, preferably whole wheat, for serving

1. Place the scrubbed clams in a large bowl and cover with cold water. Refrigerate for at least an hour or overnight (this helps remove any excess grit from the clams).

2. Heat the butter in a large pot over medium heat. Add the shallots and garlic; cook, stirring, until slightly softened, about 3 minutes. Add the red pepper flakes and cook 1 minute more. Stir in the wine and increase the heat to high. Let the wine bubble until reduced by half, about 2 minutes.

3. Add the clams and peas. Cover and cook on high heat, stirring once or twice, until the clams are beginning to open, 3 to 4 minutes. Stir in the pea shoots; cover and cook until all the clams are opened and the pea shoots are wilted, 1 to 2 minutes. Stir in the chopped mint. Serve the clam mixture and juices over hot couscous.

What Else?

- For a more classic pasta with clam sauce, serve this over cooked linguine. You can even skip the peas and pea shoots, and substitute parsley for the mint if you want to keep it very traditional.

- I honestly can't taste the difference between whole wheat and regular couscous, so I always choose whole wheat. But you can choose whichever you like best.

- If you don't want to use wine, substitute clam juice and a good squeeze of fresh lemon juice.

- You can use the larger cherrystone clams if you'd rather. I always choose littlenecks because I've got it in my head that they are sweeter. But my cousin insists they are not, and that with cherrystones, you get more clam for the buck.

HONEY-ROASTED CARROT SALAD WITH ARUGULA AND ALMONDS

The sweetest little carrots start appearing in the farmers' market in June, and I have a particular affection for the thumb-size, pale orange roots. They remind me of those few childhood years when my parents gave over nearly the entirety of our .6-acre Brooklyn backyard to cultivate a vegetable garden.

My dad spent the winters in the dark basement with his seedlings under purplish grow lights, coddling pale green shoots that he'd plant when the weather turned fine and warm.

Optimistically, my parents planted many slightly haphazard rows of tomatoes and eggplant, cucumbers, radishes, carrots, potatoes, lettuce, raspberries, blueberries, strawberries, and sweet corn. Most of it never came up (the corn was really pushing it). But just like in the classic children's book, *The Carrot Seed*, the carrots did come up. We pulled them from the ground while they were still in their infancy, and ate them rinsed under the garden hose, still warm from the ground.

Now when I see bunches of tiny, newly dug carrots at the farmers' market, I always buy them.

And even if they aren't quite as sweet as those homegrown carrots from summertimes past (and they never are), I can use them to make something good to eat, like this lovely, mellow salad. Roasting the carrots condenses their gentle flavor, making them rich and caramelized, a process I encourage by brushing them with a little honey. When they are soft and browned, I toss them with almonds for crunch and arugula for a pleasing bitter contrast. I won't wax poetic and pretend that a bite of my roasted carrot salad brings me back to my childhood, standing in the garden in muddy sneakers, carrots in hand. No, that moment is for that one-in-a-hundred carrot that happens maybe every few years.

[CONTINUED]

But my ongoing search means that I get to eat a lot of carrot salads, and this is easily one of the best. It's a simple yet spot-on combination that makes me happy every time I whip one up.

Serves 4

FOR THE SALAD

1 pound carrots (about 5 medium), trimmed, peeled,
    and cut into 1/2-inch rounds
1 1/2 tablespoons plus 2 teaspoons extra-virgin olive oil
1/2 teaspoon plus 1 large pinch kosher salt
1/4 teaspoon freshly ground black pepper
2 teaspoons honey
1/4 cup sliced almonds
2 bunches arugula (about 8 cups)

FOR THE VINAIGRETTE

1 1/2 teaspoons freshly squeezed lemon juice
1/2 teaspoon kosher salt
1/2 teaspoon freshly ground black pepper
1/4 cup extra-virgin olive oil

1. Preheat the oven to 400°F. In a large bowl, toss together the carrots, 1 1/2 tablespoons oil, 1/2 teaspoon salt, and 1/4 teaspoon pepper. Spread the carrots in an even layer on a large baking sheet. Roast, stirring occasionally, for 25 minutes.

2. Meanwhile, in a separate bowl, whisk together the honey, the remaining 2 teaspoons oil, 1 teaspoon water, and a large pinch of salt. Toss the almonds with 1 1/2 teaspoons of the honey mixture and spread them on a small baking sheet.

3. Transfer the almonds to the oven; at the same time, pour the remaining honey mixture over the carrots. Roast until the carrots are tender and caramelized and the nuts are dark golden, 5 to 7 minutes. Let the nuts and carrots cool completely.

4. Make the vinaigrette: Whisk together the lemon juice, salt, and pepper. Whisk in the oil until incorporated.

5. In a large bowl, toss together the arugula, carrots, and almonds. Add the vinaigrette and toss well to combine.

What Else?

- I once made this with Meyer lemons in the vinaigrette and it was marvelous— mellower and sweeter tasting than the original recipe, but very wonderful in its own way.

- Pistachios make a colorful substitute for the almonds.

- The flavors here are sweet and mellow, including the vinaigrette. If you'd like to tart it up, add a teaspoon or two of sharp Dijon mustard to the dressing. You'll probably have to take down the salt and lemon to balance things out (just warning you).

A Dish by Another Name

- For Honey-Roasted Butternut Squash Salad with Arugula and Almonds, sub-stitute 3/4-ish-inch chunks of peeled squash for the carrots. It's an amazing variation, just perfect for Thanksgiving or any autumnal salad craving.

GREEN PEACH SALAD WITH LIME AND BASIL

So simple, so clean, so fresh tasting, this elegant salad is just the thing to make when you've gone a little crazy at the farmers' market. You know, when you talked yourself into buying bushels of peaches in a heartfelt attempt to make pie . . . but then realized you'd need to make about four pies to use them all up.

For this dish, take the hardest, greenest, least ripe peaches of the bunch, slice them up, and eat them for dinner in a salad that is tart-sweet, light, and much more complex than the short list of ingredients would lead you to believe. That's because of the green peaches, which add a lively, fruity flavor with a fennel-like undertone that's completely unexpected. If you're not the sweet-toothed type, you might like this citrusy salad even better than pie. I might not agree, but I'll be happy to share a bowl of it with you nonetheless.

1 teaspoon freshly squeezed lime juice

1/4 teaspoon kosher salt

1/8 teaspoon freshly ground black pepper

4 teaspoons extra-virgin olive oil

1 pound green peaches (2 large or 4 small), pitted and thinly sliced

2 1/2 tablespoons thinly sliced basil leaves

Serves 4

In a bowl, whisk together the lime juice, salt, and pepper. Whisk in the oil. Add the peaches and basil and toss to combine.

What Else?

- If you can get green mango, you can use it here in place of the peaches. It makes a more savory salad, but just as mouthwatering.

- Ripe peaches work reasonably well, too, though you might have to increase the lime juice to adjust for the extra sweetness.

- Slivers of prosciutto are nice mixed in, and make this salad into lunch, served with thick slices of crusty toast slathered with olive oil.

- If you dice the peaches instead of slicing them, this becomes like salsa. Use it as a dip for chips or to top grilled fish. It's excellent.

WHOLE WHEAT PIZZA WITH THE VERY FIRST CHERRY TOMATOES, OLIVES, AND TUNA

I learned how to make pizza from Andrew Feinberg of Franny's restaurant in Brooklyn, when I was assigned to write a series of articles about him for a now defunct *New York Times* Dining Section column called "The Chef."

When Andrew and his wife Francine Stephens opened Franny's, Andrew had never made a pizza before. He learned how to make the dough from books and a lot of trial and error. "Lots of error," Francine always says when she tells the story of the restaurant's opening.

The first pies were like cardboard, with Andrew rolling the dough out with a rolling pin. She says, "I'm surprised anyone came back after that first week."

But the people did come back, and the pies improved until they became arguably some of the best in a city full of great pizza—with a slow-rising crust that is bubbly, singed in all the right spots, full of aromatic yeasty flavor, and shatteringly crisp.

The best part, for home cooks, is that you really can make a version of this fantastic pizza at home. Andrew and I came up with a technique of baking, then broiling the pizzas, which is surprisingly successful in a normal home range. Sure, in Andrew's 800°F wood-fired oven, the pizzas cook in about two minutes. At home, it takes about six. But the charred, crackling crusts are very similar in texture and flavor.

This is my version of Andrew's pie. I use a little whole wheat flour (25 percent to be exact) in the crust, just to bump up the fiber content and to give the crust a deeper, nuttier flavor. It's so good that we make pizza at home at least a few times a month, even though Franny's is only two blocks from our house. Andrew's pizza might be better at the restaurant, but at home we never have to wait for a table. And that counts for a lot.

FOR THE DOUGH

1⅛ teaspoons active dry yeast (half a ¼-ounce packet)

1 tablespoon plus 1 teaspoon kosher salt

3 cups all-purpose flour, plus additional for dusting

1 cup whole wheat flour

Olive oil, for coating the bowl

FOR THE PIZZA

6 garlic cloves, thinly sliced

Dried oregano, for sprinkling

Red pepper flakes, for sprinkling

1 cup good-quality tuna in oil, flaked

18 cherry tomatoes, halved

6 tablespoons pitted kalamata olives, halved lengthwise

Olive oil, for drizzling

Coarse sea salt, for sprinkling

3 tablespoons thinly sliced fresh basil

1. To make the dough, combine the yeast and 1¼ cups warm water in the bowl of an electric mixer. Let the mixture sit until foamy, about 5 minutes. Add the salt and flours. Mix on medium-high speed until the dough comes together, adding more warm water as needed. You should not knead the dough, but do mix it until the dough just becomes supple and smooth. Place the dough in an oil-coated bowl and cover loosely with plastic wrap. Transfer to the re-frigerator and let rise at least 24 hours or up to 3 days. When ready to use the dough, divide it into 3 equal-size pieces. Shape the dough into balls. Let it sit at room temperature at least 30 minutes before using; this will make a big difference in the ease with which your dough will stretch to pizzaworthy size.

2. To make the pizza, preheat the oven to 500°F. Arrange an oven rack in the top third of the oven. Place a pizza stone on the rack. Let it heat for 1 hour. Or use an overturned baking dish and preheat for 30 minutes.

3. Turn a large baking sheet upside down and dust the surface with flour. Place a dough ball on a clean, lightly floured surface; dust the top of the

[CONTINUED]

dough with additional flour. Use your fingertips to flatten the dough into a round. Holding the dough in front of you like a steering wheel (with your hands at 10 o'clock and 2 o'clock), rotate the dough several times between your hands, stretching it slightly as you do so. Try to maintain as even a thickness as possible, with the outermost edges of the dough slightly thicker. Continue, working carefully around thin patches of dough to ensure that it does not tear, until you have a 12-ish-inch round. (Or use a rolling pin to roll out the dough.)

4. Carefully set the dough down upon the floured baking sheet. Patch any tears or holes in the dough. Working quickly, scatter the dough with a third of the sliced garlic, a pinch of dried oregano, and a pinch of red pepper flakes. Scatter a third of the tuna, 12 tomato slices, and 2 tablespoons olives.

5. Jiggle the pizza gently on the pan to make sure it is not sticking. Slide the pizza directly onto the hot stone; make sure to start holding the pan at the stone's back end so that the entire pizza will fit. Drizzle the pizza generously with oil.

6. Cook the pizza until the underside is golden and the top is firm, 3 minutes. Turn off the oven and turn on the broiler. Broil the pizza until golden, crisp, and a bit blistery and charred in places, 1 to 4 minutes (watch it carefully to see that it does not burn).

7. Use tongs to slide the pizza to a large platter. Drizzle it with oil and salt; garnish with basil.

8. Repeat the cooking process with the remaining dough balls and toppings.

What Else?

- If you have one of those ovens with the broiler on a separate drawer on the bottom, don't use the broiling method. Just leave the pizza in the 500°F oven until it is crisp and golden brown all over. It will take 8 to 15 minutes.

- The dough recipe was originally created using entirely all-purpose flour, so if you would rather cleave to the original, go ahead. You might have to reduce the water slightly. Go by feel; you want a slightly sticky, floppy dough.

- Yes, you really do have to refrigerate this dough overnight; the long, slow rise helps develop its yeasty, full flavor. It would taste bland if you let it rise quickly at room temperature.

- You can make the dough ahead and freeze balls of it. It will defrost in about 2 hours if left on the kitchen counter. Or pull it out in the morning and let it defrost all day in the fridge. It will be perfect come dinnertime. We always have some on hand.

- There are so many ways to top this dough, I could probably devote an entire book to it, if not at least a chapter. The short version is to just use your favorite combination of ingredients, because if you think it sounds good on a pizza, chances are it will taste good on a pizza. A word of caution: Be restrained about how much stuff you add to the crust. You want to embellish it without weighing it down. A light touch here is essential.

  One thing to keep in mind is that if you want a tomato sauce, it's best to use an uncooked sauce of pureed canned tomatoes rather than a cooked pasta-type sauce, which gets too jammy tasting and loses its freshness. Add the sauce to the pie after you've transferred it to the pizza stone, or things could get sticky and messy. Then for the classic pizza pie, quickly scatter on some sliced fresh mozzarella, dried oregano, and a slick of olive oil. Your Margherita will be ready in minutes.

BUCKWHEAT PANCAKES WITH SLICED PEACHES AND CARDAMOM CREAM SYRUP

One of the newest farms to join the market this past year is the grains folks at Cayuga Organics. I love their products, and not just because they are local, but because they're so much fresher than what you get at even the fanciest gourmet market. While freshness isn't a huge issue for things like bleached white flour, it is extremely important with whole grains and whole grain flours, which can go rancid really quickly. And even a slight rancidity can make whole grains and whole grain baked goods taste bitter before they actually smell off.

Because of this access, I've been experimenting with a range of different whole grain flours, and have found that I absolutely adore the complex, winey nuttiness of buckwheat flour. It's traditionally used in blinis, but since I don't make blinis very often (sadly because I don't serve caviar very often), I decided to try it in a regular old pancake, the kind I make for breakfast on the weekends. Since I don't bother using yeast, the flavor isn't as complex as a blini, but the buttermilk gives it a nice fresh tang and the honey lends a little sweetness that makes these pancakes wonderful on their own, should you choose to forgo any syrupy distractions.

If you are interested in syrup, however, please try this oddball, creamy, exotic-scented, and utterly divine cardamom cream syrup at least once. I can't really tell you how I came up with it other than to say I like the combination of cardamom with juicy ripe peaches, which I planned to scatter over the pancakes before serving. And I like cardamom cream cakes, which I ate on a brief trip to Sweden when I was briefly married to a Swede (a man, not a vegetable). Come to think of it, they grow buckwheat in Sweden, and I'm sure my subconscious was aware of this as I made breakfast that day. So there you have it: Cardamom, cream, peaches, and buckwheat are a natural—okay, a plausible—combination.

In any case, it all works and tastes delicious, no matter how you connect the dots.

FOR THE CARDAMOM CREAM SYRUP

1 tablespoon cardamom pods, crushed

1/3 cup sugar

1/4 cup heavy cream

Pinch kosher salt

FOR THE PANCAKES

3/4 cup all-purpose flour

1/2 cup buckwheat flour

1/2 cup whole wheat flour

2 teaspoons baking powder

1 teaspoon baking soda

1/2 teaspoon kosher salt

1 large egg, lightly beaten

1 tablespoon honey

2 cups buttermilk or plain yogurt, more as needed

3 tablespoons unsalted butter, melted, more as needed

Sliced fresh peaches, for serving

1. In a small saucepan, combine the cardamom, sugar, and 1/3 cup water. Bring to a simmer and cook until the sugar has fully dissolved, about 5 minutes. Stir in the cream and salt and let it bubble gently for 2 minutes. Let the syrup cool completely; strain.

2. Make the pancakes: In a large bowl, whisk together the flours, baking powder, baking soda, and salt. In a separate bowl, whisk together the egg and honey; whisk in the buttermilk or yogurt and melted butter. Form a well in the dry ingredients. Pour the wet ingredients into the well and stir until just combined.

3. Melt some butter on a griddle or in a large skillet over medium-high heat. Working in batches, spoon 1/4-cup dollops of batter onto the griddle. Cook the pancakes until bubbles form on the surface and the edges

[CONTINUED]

begin to set, 2 to 3 minutes. Flip and cook until golden, 1 to 2 minutes more. Cook additional pancakes, adding more butter to the skillet if necessary. Serve the pancakes hot, topped with the cardamom syrup and peaches.

What Else?

- We make these pancakes all year round, so please don't wait for peach season. They are lovely on their own, sans fruit, served with regular old maple syrup in place of the fancy cardamom syrup I write about here. In that case, you could even add a pinch of ground cardamom to the pancake batter so that you don't miss out on the fragrant spice.

- If you don't have buckwheat flour, you can use all whole wheat.

- For a richer pancake, I like to stir in sour cream in place of the buttermilk. Actually, to be honest, I'll use whatever I've got, be it sour cream, buttermilk, or plain whole milk yogurt. All of them have the right acidity level to make these pancakes featherlight, so feel free to choose your favorite. Or stir together a fridge-cleaning combination.

OBSESSIVE TWICE-BAKED SOUR CHERRY PIE

Truth be told, I was only 90 percent happy with the sour cherry pie recipe I published one summer in my Good Appetite column in the *New York Times*. The crust, a twice-baked beauty using a technique I learned from White House pastry chef Bill Yosses, was terrific—crisp, buttery, able to stand up to all those sweet cherry juices. And the filling, made with Minute tapioca (aka instant tapioca), was shining, clear, and just firm enough. My only beef was with the filling texture. Instead of being perfectly smooth, it still had tiny little tapioca beads floating in it, like a cherry-flavored tapioca pudding. You'd barely notice them if you weren't looking. But I *was* looking, and once I found them, they bugged me. And a few of the tiny tapioca pearls that ended up sitting on top of the cherries, peeking through the crust, baked up with a slight sandy crunch. My friends and family think I'm nuts, by the way, but so be it. During the blink-your-eyes-and-you'll-miss-it sour cherry season, I want my once-a-year sour cherry pie to be perfect.

Thus began my obsessive cherry pie experimentation. I wanted to change up the starch so the filling would be clear, tasteless, and perfectly smooth.

Having made pies with both flour and cornstarch in the past, I rejected those; the flour has a pasty flavor and the cornstarch isn't quite as clear as I was looking for (though it's close and it's definitely my second favorite thickener).

But two starches I hadn't tried were potato starch and tapioca starch (aka tapioca flour). I had read glowing reports about their marvelous thickening power in fruit pies. I was gravely disappointed in both. The tapioca was cloudy and had a bitter aftertaste. (We ate it anyway.) The potato starch was also cloudy, pasty, and gave me cherry soup in a crust. (We ate part of it, then had to toss it after the whole pie kind of dissolved into an unappetizing

[CONTINUED]

mush). I read somewhere that potato starch can break down when boiled, and perhaps that is what happened to me.

One thing I found interesting was that tapioca starch was not just ground-up instant tapioca pearls. Tapioca pearls, the kind used to make pudding, are treated to become more stable. The starch is a less processed product, but also less predictable in its thickening power. This might be why I had such problems with my pie, whereas I've heard reports that other people's pies are just swell using the stuff. You can't count on it.

In the end, I decided to grind up 2 tablespoons instant tapioca in a clean coffee grinder until it turned to powder. (I had tried it in the food processor and while it did make the pearls smaller, it didn't turn them to powder the way the grinder did.) Then I mixed the powder into the cherries.

The result? The filling is clear, flavorless, glossy, and thickened without being firmly set or gloppy (you could use a little more if you like your pie completely set). I also used a teensy bit of lard in the crust to make it extra flaky.

In a word: Yum. Or possibly: Insane. Either shoe is a likely fit.

FOR THE CRUST

Serves 8

1¾ cups plus 2 tablespoons all-purpose flour

⅜ teaspoon kosher salt

13 tablespoons unsalted butter, chilled and cut into pieces

2 tablespoons lard, chilled (or use more butter)

3 to 6 tablespoons ice water, as needed

FOR THE FILLING

2 to 3 tablespoons instant tapioca (more if you like it very set, less if you don't mind a little thickened juice)

1 cup granulated sugar (or more if you like a sweeter pie)

¼ teaspoon ground cinnamon

2 pounds sour cherries (about 6 cups), rinsed and pitted

1 tablespoon kirsch or brandy

3 tablespoons heavy cream

Demerara (raw) sugar, for sprinkling

1. First, make the dough. In the bowl of a food processor, pulse together the flour and salt just to combine. Add the butter and lard and pulse until lima bean–size pieces form. Add the water 1 tablespoon at a time and pulse until the mixture just comes together. Pat the dough into 2 discs, one using two-thirds of the dough, the other using one-third of the dough (weigh it if you have a kitchen scale; one disc should be about 12 ounces, the other 6 ounces). Wrap the discs in plastic and refrigerate at least 1 hour (and up to 3 days) before rolling out and baking.

2. Preheat the oven to 425°F. Place the large disc on a lightly floured surface and roll it into a 12-inch circle about 3/8 inch thick. Transfer the dough to a 9-inch pie plate. Line the dough with foil and weigh it down with pie weights (I use pennies, but dry beans or rice will also work). Bake until the crust is light golden brown, about 30 minutes.

3. While the piecrust is baking, prepare the filling: Using a coffee or spice grinder, grind the tapioca to a fine powder. In a small bowl, combine the tapioca with the granulated sugar and cinnamon. Place the cherries in a bowl and add the sugar and tapioca mixture. Drizzle in the kirsch or brandy and toss gently to combine.

4. When the piecrust is ready, transfer it to a wire rack to cool slightly and reduce the temperature to 375°F. Remove the foil and pie weights and scrape the cherry filling into the piecrust.

5. Place the smaller disc of dough on a lightly floured surface and roll it 3/8 inch thick. Use a round cookie cutter (or several round cookie cutters of different sizes) to cut out circles of dough. Arrange the dough circles on top of the cherry filling.

6. Brush the dough circles with cream and sprinkle the top of the pie generously with Demerara sugar. Bake until the crust is dark golden brown and the filling begins to bubble, 50 minutes to 1 hour. Transfer the pie to a wire rack to cool for at least 2 hours, allowing the filling to set up before serving.

What Else?

- If you would rather simply use cornstarch, use 3 tablespoons for 2 pounds of cherries. This will give you a lightly set filling that's still a little runny when you cut it, which is just how I like it.

- The twice-baked crust is amazing, and it's now my go-to technique for any fruit pie because it stays crisp despite all the glorious juices. So please try it with any fruit pie you feel like making.

- After years of using a hairpin to pit cherries, I finally broke down and bought a nifty cherry pitter—the large boxy kind where you pour in the cherries and then punch a lever to remove the pit. I use it once a year during cherry season, but I use it hard, pitting cherries for pies, jams, sauces, and my now famous-among-my-friends maraschino cherries. At under $50, it's a hugely worthwhile investment that any cherry lover should consider.

Summer

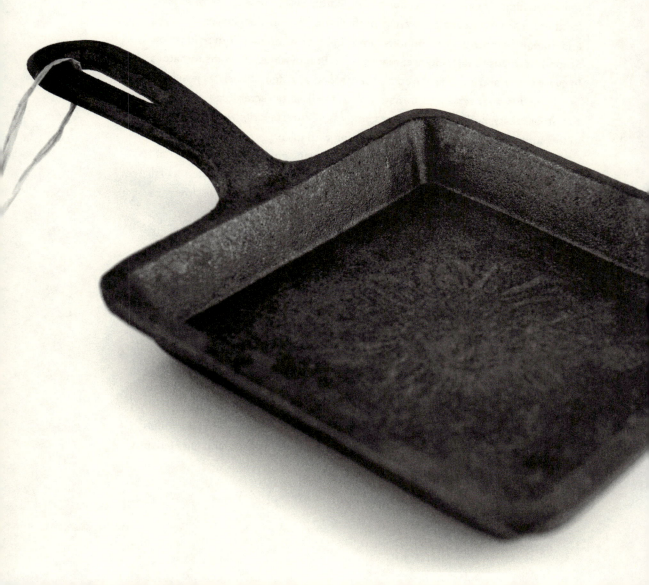

The first day of summer might technically fall in June, but for me, the season doesn't really begin until mid-July when fat, ripe heirloom tomatoes make their way to the farmers' market in earnest.

And by earnest, I don't mean a few meager boxes of red and yellow cherry tomatoes hiding near the checkout scales, hardly visible unless you're looking for them. Earnest means a dizzying profusion of scarlet beefsteaks, mini red and orange teardrops, and luminous lumpy heirlooms ranging from mild yellow Striped Germans to tart, intense, mauve-hued Brandywines. It means tomatoes in every shape and size, displayed on every stand as ostentatiously as jewels.

It means gazpacho and tomato salad, fresh salsa, scrambled eggs with tomatoes, zesty, herby tomato sauces, and my all-time favorite way to eat lunch in the summer: a tomato sandwich, dripping with juice.

I get so carried away in the presence of so many gorgeous tomatoes that I always buy too many, lugging them home until my shoulders threaten to fall out of their sockets and my arms are ringed with nasty red furrows from the bag handles.

Of course, tomatoes aren't the only culprits weighing down those bags. Summer is a season of bounty, and bounty is heavy. It's ripe, nectar laden, and cumbersome. It smacks against my legs on the long walk home.

Before Daniel and I had Dahlia, every summer farmers' market trip was combined with a nice, humid, sweaty run, since my local market is adjacent to Prospect Park. I'd jog the half-mile to the park, around the (smaller) loop (another 2.2 miles), and then shop the overloaded stands, celebrating the abundance by buying as much as I could possibly schlep, using the bulging bags as weights to do bicep curls on the walk home. It beats the gym and got me something good to eat all week long.

Now summer trips to the farmers' market have become just as much about entertaining our two-year-old as about tomatoes, melons, and juicy, crisp cucumbers.

Although we bring Dahlia to the market with us all year long, summer is the most fun for her, and by extension, fun for us to be there with her. The balmy weather means we can linger and let her charm the farmers with a shy hello, which always seems to be enough to win all kinds of little gifts—a fuzzy purple chive flower, a sweet carrot, a tiny yellow plum.

Then, when the stroller is loaded and we cannot cram another slim green bean into the bags, we settle onto a grassy patch next to the statue of James Stranahan, one of the founders of the park.

There's always a posse of kids and their still-caffeinating parents there, running around and around the statue (the kids, that is), taking turns being the chaser and the chased.

Dahlia is happy to sit on the side with her tiny friend Alice, eating cherry tomatoes and blueberries and sometimes shucking the corn. Dahlia learned this most helpful skill from Alice, or really, from Alice's mother, Anna, and she's taken to it with gusto: ripping off the green peels and gently pulling the silks, one shimmering thread at a time, taking bites of the corn as she goes. By the time we get home, the corns are perfectly husked and missing a bite or two, a casualty I'm happy to endure, given the joy it gives her.

Also in my bags to unpack are piles of peaches and nectarines, most of which get eaten plain, over the sink to catch the honeyed drips as they roll off my fingers. Sometimes I'll slice them up for fruit salad or as a juicy topping for buckwheat pancakes (page 186). And every summer, at least once, I'll make some variation on peach ice cream (page 220), trying to recapture a fleeting flavor I remember from childhood.

Ditto the apricots, which I rarely cook, instead enjoying their tart, jammy flesh in small nibbles, one ripe fruit after the other. The thing about apricots is that their window for ripeness is short and it seems to happen all at once. July is the month of apricot feast or famine, when I find myself either stuffing myself with the speckled, amber fruit or waiting impatiently for the next batch to soften.

There is no need to wait to eat the berries, which I can unpack and devour on the spot. Raspberries are my favorite; I buy them every Saturday morning for a late breakfast, coated in a little heavy cream or whole milk yogurt and sprinkled with glittery Demerara sugar. Dahlia likes the blueberries best, and whatever tiny purple orbs make it home from the market before she gets a chance to eat the whole pint will get nibbled into oblivion by the end of the weekend—unless I am clever about hiding an extra pint in the fridge to turn into tea cake (page 217) or one of Daniel's purple smoothies.

Summer isn't all about juicy fruit and ripe tomatoes (which are botanically a fruit and legally a vegetable, in case you were curious). Vegetables abound, especially plump, seedy ones like cucumbers, summer squash, eggplant, and zucchini, and fleshy, sweet ones such as bell peppers, mushrooms, and corn. The hardest part is choosing which to buy, since they all look so glossy and lovely, piled neatly into wooden boxes and milk crates. Usually I just get them all.

In contrast to what seems to be the trend in food magazines, I don't typically grill my summer vegetables, even when I've got the coals going hot and strong to char some meat. I prefer summer vegetables prepared simply, in colorful salads with piquant dressings (Shaved Zucchini and Avocado Salad with Green Goddess Dressing, page 244 and Shaved Fennel Salad with Parmesan and Orange Zest, page 204) or, perhaps strangely for this time of year, roasted in the oven (Roasted Pepper and Celery Leaf Crostini, page 260, and Fresh Corn Polenta with Roasted Ratatouille and Ricotta, page 268). Mostly this is because I'm better at roasting and salad making than I am at grilling vegetables. Meat is forgiving. As long as you don't overcook it, it usually tastes great just thrown onto the fire. Not so with vegetables, which need finessing to turn out burnished, glistening, and sweet tasting.

No matter what I cook or how I cook it (or not cook it, as is often the case with hot-weather eating), summer food is about ease and freshness and bounty; it's about cocktails and dinner on the deck at dusk, after Dahlia is in bed but before it gets dark enough to light the citronella candles. And yes, summer wouldn't be summer without mosquitoes, who probably look forward to supping on me as much as I look forward to that first heirloom tomato. And that is an awful lot.

JULY

CANTALOUPE AND YOGURT SOUP WITH TOASTED CUMIN SALT

I came up with this cool, refreshing soup on one of the sweatiest, stickiest, steamiest lunchtimes of summer. It was the kind of day when, despite our valiant air conditioner's best efforts, it was just too darn hot to do *anything* at all, let alone chew. Whatever I had for lunch would have to be blended into liquid submission, and my first thought was to make an icy fruit smoothie.

Oddly for me, though, I didn't feel like my usual honeyed ice-yogurt-fruit mix. Maybe it was the heat, but I was craving salt, something potato chip-salty, in sippable form.

I briefly contemplated gazpacho. The spicy flavors seemed right, but all that vegetable chopping was just too much work.

Then I remembered another savory blender creation, a bracing Indian yogurt drink called a lassi that I love to order in Indian restaurants but never think to make at home. Frothed up from yogurt, salt, ice, and sometimes lemon juice and/or cumin, it's salty, filling, and ridiculously easy, a perfect summer lunch.

I whirled one together and took a taste. It was cold and zippy enough to quell my cravings, but it still needed a little something to make it totally satisfying.

Maybe it was my fruit smoothie associations pulling hard, but it seemed to me that it could use a sweet element to balance out the yogurt tanginess. I poked around in the fridge, and unearthed a bowl of cut-up cantaloupe and half a jalapeño left over from some recent guacamole making. I threw them both in the blender bowl, hoping to hit a range of sweet, tart, salty, spicy flavors.

I poured my new creation into my smoothie glass and took a sip. It was earthy from the cumin, fruity, and very creamy, with a gentle bite from the pepper. It was far too heady and complex to sip through a straw, so I moved it to a bowl and took up a spoon.

As I ate, I fantasized about serving it at my next summer dinner party as a nuanced, ten-minute first course, maybe gussied up in my prettiest glass bowls to show off the melon color, topped with some crunchy cumin salt.

I suppose I could have even done the same thing for lunch, except the blender was empty and my belly was full. Happily, there were many weeks of summer left, which meant many sticky, sweaty days and all the good liquid food that went with them.

Serves 4 to 6

2 pounds peeled and cubed cantaloupe (8 cups)
1 cup plain yogurt
1/2 to 1 jalapeño, to taste, seeded and finely chopped
2 teaspoons freshly squeezed lemon juice
1/2 teaspoon kosher salt
1 teaspoon whole cumin seed
2 teaspoons coarse sea salt

1. Combine the cantaloupe, yogurt, jalapeño, lemon juice, and salt in a blender and puree until smooth. Pour into a bowl, cover tightly with plastic wrap, and chill for 1 hour.

2. In a small skillet over medium heat, toast the cumin seeds until fragrant, about 1 minute. Pour into a mortar and pestle and add the coarse sea salt. Pound the mixture a few times until the cumin seeds are lightly crushed. If you don't have a mortar and pestle, put the cumin and salt onto a cutting board and either smack it with the side of a heavy cleaver or knife, or roll over them with a rolling pin or the side of a wine bottle.

3. To serve, ladle the soup into individual bowls. Garnish with the cumin salt.

What Else?

- Here's the place where I'd usually write about how I'd substitute something for the yogurt to make this soup Daniel-appropriate. In this case, I wouldn't bother. It's not his thing. He isn't a huge cantaloupe fan, espe-

[CONTINUED]

cially not liquid cantaloupe. I have, on occasion, added a few surreptitious cubes to his morning smoothie, and he is never pleased.

- If you don't feel like making the cumin salt, you don't have to. Just use regular flaky sea salt mixed with a little powdered cumin or some of that Turkish or Aleppo pepper that I'm sure I've talked you into tracking down by now.

- Other dense-fleshed melons, such as honeydew or Galia melons, work well here as a cantaloupe substitution. Watermelon does not. It's too porous and watery, and makes a bland soup.

- And while I'm thinking about it, you might notice I don't have a single watermelon recipe in this book. This is because my favorite way to eat watermelon doesn't need a recipe: Just slice it up, sprinkle with sea salt, and gobble it up. Simple and perfect, it's the essence of summer eating.

SHRIMP SCAMPI WITH PERNOD AND FENNEL FRONDS

I've gotten complacent when it comes to shrimp cookery. Out of the dozens of methods possible for cooking the crustacean, I've reduced it to two, which fall along a seasonal divide.

In winter, I roast them until caramelized and golden; in summer, I sauté them with garlic, scampi style.

Not that I make the same two dishes over and over. I keep the techniques consistent, and change up the flavorings to match my mood and the contents of my fridge.

For example, this licorice-scented scampi is the love child of a bag of shrimp and a shock of wandering, feathery fennel fronds that met in the fridge while waiting for me to figure out what to make for dinner. When I opened the fridge and noticed their intimate proximity, the dish seemed destined to be.

So I married them in the pan, anointing the union with butter for creaminess, crushed red pepper for heat, and Pernod to play up the anise flavor of the fennel. I have to say, it's one of the happiest pairings to ever end up on my dinner plate.

You'll notice I don't use the fennel bulbs here. I could have, slicing them thinly and caramelizing them in butter before adding the shrimp. But in the end I decided to keep things simple and pure between fronds and seafood. After all, three's a crowd, even in a sauté pan.

Serves 4 to 6

3 tablespoons unsalted butter
2 garlic cloves, minced
1/3 cup dry white wine
2 tablespoons Pernod
3/4 teaspoon kosher salt, or to taste

[CONTINUED]

Pinch crushed red pepper flakes

2 pounds large shrimp, shelled

2 tablespoons fresh, finely minced fennel fronds (save the bulbs for
    snacking or for the fennel salad on page 204)

Freshly squeezed juice of ½ lemon

1. In a large skillet over medium heat, melt the butter. Add the garlic and
   cook, stirring, until fragrant, about 1 minute. Add the wine and Pernod,
   salt, and red pepper flakes. Bring to a simmer. Let the mixture reduce by
   half, about 2 minutes.

2. Add the shrimp and cook, stirring, until they just turn pink, 2 to 4 minutes
   depending on their size. Stir in the fennel fronds and lemon juice. Serve
   with crusty bread.

What Else?

Scampi is such an adaptable recipe because the combination of butter, garlic,
and wine makes anything taste good. So, to that end, here are a few of my
favorite variations:

- Skip the Pernod and use Cognac or more white wine.

- Any fresh, floppy, soft herb can step into the fennel fronds' shoes. Parsley
  is classic, mint is refreshing, sage is musky, basil is summery, cilantro is
  citrusy, anise hyssop is exotic, chervil is licorice-ish, and a combination
  might just blow your mind.

- Chunks of fish or scallops or even chicken can replace the shrimp if you're
  not feeling shrimpy.

- A pinch of Turkish or Aleppo red pepper is a nice substitute for the more
  pedestrian red pepper flakes, adding a fruity, smoky note.

- Lime juice is nice sometimes instead of the lemon. To bump up the citrus flavor of either lemon or lime, you can also grate in some fresh zest, which zips things up nicely, especially given the butter quotient here.

- If you like it aromatic, try adding a pinch of garam masala or ground cumin to the butter.

- Sometimes I throw some cubed tomatoes into the pan along with the shrimp. If you do this, you'll need more salt and pepper to season everything properly.

SHAVED FENNEL SALAD WITH PARMESAN AND ORANGE ZEST

Naturally I'd never write a recipe calling for just the fennel fronds (Shrimp Scampi with Pernod and Fennel Fronds, page 201) without having a plan for the bulb itself . . . would I?

Well, to tell you the truth, when I hacked off the feathery fronds for my scampi, I had no idea how I'd make use of the sweet, crunchy bulb.

I knew I'd do something because *a*) I love fennel, and *b*) who buys fennel bulbs just for the fronds? I'd get kicked out of the Imaginary Society of Commonsense Food Writers if I published a recipe like that ("2 tablespoons chopped fennel fronds, discard the bulbs").

Of course there is nothing wrong with just munching the fennel as a little predinner snack while you mince through their greens. I do it all the time. But when I want something more substantial from my bulb, I make a shaved fennel salad.

I know that one can make fennel salad from chopped fennel or sliced fennel, or some other fennel deconstruction method. But ever since I discovered the joys of running a halved bulb over the razor edge of a mandoline so it fluffs into a tangle of feathery white leaves, I've never gone back to the knife.

For this salad, I kept things simple, adding orange zest and juice to play up the sweet anise flavor of the fennel, along with a little vinegar for brightness and lots of aged Parmesan cheese, because I always add cheese to salads when Daniel isn't joining me. It was crisp, refreshing, savory, and just filling enough, which is exactly what I want from a light summer lunch.

2 large fennel bulbs, trimmed and outer layers removed

1/2 teaspoon finely grated orange zest

2 tablespoons freshly squeezed orange juice

1 tablespoon red wine vinegar

Serves 2 for lunch or
4 as an appetizer

½ teaspoon kosher salt

½ teaspoon freshly ground black pepper

3 tablespoons extra-virgin olive oil (use your best stuff)

2 ounces Parmesan cheese (optional)

1. Cut each fennel bulb in half lengthwise. Using a mandoline-type tool or very sharp knife, thinly shave the fennel. Transfer to a large bowl

2. In a small bowl, whisk together the orange zest, orange juice, vinegar, salt, and pepper. Whisk in the oil. Pour the dressing over the fennel and toss well.

3. Working over the salad bowl, use a vegetable peeler to shave the cheese into thin curls. Toss the salad gently once more and serve.

What Else?

• Yes, go ahead and leave off the cheese. I just added it because I was eating this for lunch by myself and that's when I like to cheese it up. If you want to vary things, blue cheese makes a pungent Parmesan substitute, while ricotta salata crumbles pleasingly into firm yet creamy chunks.

• If you want to take this in a sweeter direction, add some thinly sliced dates to the mix.

• If you haven't defronded your fennel to make scampi, you can use the fronds here as a garnish.

• You can substitute a lesser quantity of lemon juice and zest for the orange. Just start with a few drops and taste as you go, adding more until the flavor pleases you.

• If you don't have a mandoline, really, go get one now. They lie perfectly flat, so they don't take up much storage space, and you can buy a Japanese

[CONTINUED]

Benriner for under $40. It makes slicing vegetables so much easier (with prettier results than you can get with a knife). And once you have one, it will tempt you into making potato chips at least once and probably a lot more often than that. (Yes, you can even bake them if you hate deep-frying.) Homemade potato chips, fried in olive oil, are heaven.

PANFRIED STRIPED BASS WITH ANCHOVY GARLIC BREAD CRUMBS AND BASIL

I have a little crush on anchovies.

Whenever I see a glass jar lined with those red-streaked, oily brown fillets, my heart leaps and I get tingly all over in that hungry-for-dinner way. I am crazy about how the little salted fish add a depth of flavor to just about anything, without necessarily tasting fishy—just intensely savory and salty, rich and deep.

They are nearly perfect on their own, but when combined with garlic and a little butter or olive oil, the combination makes me swoon.

Here's what I like to do: Heat a little oil or butter in a pan, then add chopped garlic and whole anchovy fillets, letting the garlic warm and turn opaque and the anchovies dissolve (which they do; you don't need to chop them). This flavorful elixir is the start of many of my favorite things to eat. And the best part is, I can whip it up in minutes from staples I always have on hand (I will break out into a nervous sweat if I'm out of anchovies or garlic, so I keep emergency supplies on hand).

One of my favorite ways to use the sauce is as a medium for browning plain bread crumbs. The crumbs get crisp and imbued with garlicky-anchovy goodness, and taste utterly wonderful, even by the handful.

I often toss the crumbs into pasta in place of grated cheese. But in this instance, I sprinkled them on top of some lightly sautéed striped bass I managed to score from the farmers' market. They added a nice, crunchy texture to the soft, velvety fish, and a piquant flavor that went well with its sweetness. And even with two fish on the plate, there was nothing fishy about it.

3 tablespoons unsalted butter

3 anchovy fillets

2 garlic cloves, finely chopped

½ cup coarse bread crumbs

Freshly ground black pepper to taste

2 tablespoons extra-virgin olive oil

Kosher salt to taste

4 (6- to 8-ounce) skin-on striped bass fillets, patted dry

Chopped fresh basil, for serving

Lemon wedges, for serving

1. Melt the butter in a large skillet over medium-high heat. Add the anchovies and cook, stirring and breaking up with a wooden spoon, until the anchovies have melted into the butter, 1 to 2 minutes. Stir in the garlic and cook for 30 seconds. Add the bread crumbs and cook until golden brown, about 2 minutes. Season with pepper. Scrape the bread crumbs into a small bowl.

2. Wipe out the pan and return it to medium-high heat. Add the oil and heat until very hot but not smoking. Season the fish with salt and pepper. Add the fish to the skillet, skin-side down. It should sizzle when it hits the pan. Cook, without moving, until the edges and sides of the fish are opaque, about 5 minutes. Carefully flip the fish and continue cooking until it is completely opaque and beginning to flake, 2 to 3 minutes more.

3. To serve, arrange the fish on individual serving plates. Scatter basil over the fillets and top with the bread crumbs. Serve with lemon wedges.

What Else?

- You can use the anchovy garlic sauce without the crumbs on pretty much anything that won't mind a pungent drizzle. Paint it on croutons for salad, spoon it over cooked fish or chicken, toss it with pasta or roasted vegetables. Once, I poured the hot sauce over a fresh mozzarella and tomato salad, where it warmed the tomatoes, releasing their flavor, and ever so slightly softened the cheese. The possibilities are infinite.

- I've used the same crumbs to top other fish fillets, as well as scallops and shrimp. The thing is to cook the fish separately, then use a heavy hand to spoon on the crumbs. Trust me, you'll want lots of them.

- In my last book, *In the Kitchen with A Good Appetite*, I wrote a recipe for pan-seared asparagus topped with fried eggs and these bread crumbs. I make it every year during asparagus season and if you love asparagus, eggs, and a crunchy bite, you will, too.

CUCUMBER AND ALMOND
SALAD WITH SHISO

One summer long ago, before I knew better than to plant herbs willy-nilly in my back garden, I stuck a purple shiso plant into the ground along with a teensy lemon balm. For a while, I luxuriated in the fact that I never had to buy those herbs again, because every year they came back even more abundantly than the summer before.

After a few seasons, lemon balm carpeted my entire yard, fighting with the violets for soil space, while the shiso poked its spiky leaves through the gaps in the rocks and took root in every flowerpot within spitting distance, from the coleus on the deck to the basil in my window box. By the time it started peeping through the mossy cracks in the brick path, I realized I'd made a mistake. These weedy plants had to go.

Daniel spent a backbreaking spring digging up all the roots, removing every tiny white tendril he could find, sifting out the black soil.

His prodigious efforts did manage to eradicate the violets (which was mostly good but a little sad, since they were beautiful for the one week they blossomed before turning leggy and ugly for the rest of the season). But the shiso and lemon balm still sprout up, perkily as ever, as soon as the weather turns fine.

Thus, I use a lot of shiso in my salads, where it adds a peppery, tangy, grassy note that I've especially come to love with cool, crunchy cucumbers. I've made many versions of cucumber shiso salad, but this one, with an Asian influence, is my current favorite. Of course that may change next summer when the shiso grows back and I play around some more. After all, if you can't beat it, eat it.

1/4 cup slivered almonds

1 pound tender-skinned Kirby cucumbers, trimmed

2 1/2 teaspoons soy sauce

Serves 4

2 teaspoons sesame oil

1 teaspoon freshly squeezed lime juice

1 tablespoon finely chopped shiso leaves

Flaky sea salt to taste

1. In a small skillet over medium-high heat, toast the almonds, shaking the pan occasionally, until golden, about 4 minutes.
2. Cut the cucumber in half lengthwise; cut each half crosswise into $\frac{1}{4}$-inch half-moons. (If your cucumbers have thick skins, you should peel them first.)
3. In a small bowl, whisk together the soy sauce, sesame oil, and lime juice. Toss the dressing with the cucumbers and almonds. Sprinkle with the shiso and salt. Serve.

What Else?

- If you've got some nice ripe tomatoes, throw them in. I do it all the time. Golden cherry tomatoes are especially tasty here, and they don't exude too much juice, which can be distracting to the folks who don't like the way the tomato water pools on the bottom of the salad bowl (I just drink it up when the bowl is otherwise empty).

- Sometimes, when I'm looking for a mellow flavor profile, I like to use extra-virgin olive oil in place of the sesame oil. It makes for a gentler salad.

- If you want a sweet burst of fruitiness, try adding some perfectly ripe sliced yellow plums. It sounds weird but it tastes great.

- In case you were curious, the lemon balm is not so good in salads. I like it as a lemonade or iced tea garnish, or steeped into simple syrup, which I often toss with sliced peaches and plums.

LAMB MERGUEZ BURGERS WITH HARISSA MAYONNAISE

There is a minimalist elegance to a good hamburger. Simply seasoned with salt and pepper and grilled to medium-rare perfection, it needs nothing more than a soft white bun to reach its meaty potential, though an assortment of tasty accoutrements (pickles, lettuce, tomatoes, ketchup, blue cheese) can only make things better—if you're the burger-topping type.

At the other end of the spectrum is my spicy lamb burger. Imbued with coriander, fennel, cayenne, and plenty of onion and garlic, it's got the same flavor profile as a merguez sausage but is shaped into a burger-patty package. When served charred on the outside and juicy within, it is bold, intense, deeply savory, and about as far from minimalist as you can get, in the best possible way.

I like to serve it in a whole wheat pita pocket swathed in harissa mayonnaise and piled high with crunchy vegetables. But the fiery, gamy flavors of chile and lamb can easily stand alone on the plate—before you come along to gobble it up.

½ teaspoon coriander seed

½ teaspoon fennel seed

1 pound ground lamb

¼ cup finely chopped onion

2 tablespoons cold unsalted butter, cut into small pieces

2 garlic cloves, finely chopped

1½ teaspoons kosher salt

1 teaspoon paprika

Pinch cayenne

Olive oil, for brushing

⅓ cup mayonnaise

1½ teaspoons harissa, or to taste

Serves 4

4 whole wheat or regular pita breads
Sliced cucumber, for serving
Sliced tomatoes, for serving
Salad greens, for serving

1. In a dry skillet over medium heat, toast the coriander seed and fennel seed until fragrant. Transfer the spices to a spice grinder and finely grind (alternatively, you can use a mortar and pestle).

2. In a large bowl, mix together the ground spices, lamb, onion, butter, garlic, salt, paprika, and cayenne until just combined. Form into 4 equal-size patties, about 3/4 inch thick.

3. Preheat a grill to medium-high. Brush the grate lightly with oil. Place the burgers on the grill. Close the cover and cook to the desired doneness, about 3 minutes per side for medium-rare. Let the burgers rest 5 minutes before serving.

4. In a small bowl, whisk together the mayonnaise and harissa; spoon into the pitas. Fill the pitas with the burgers, cucumber, tomatoes, and greens.

What Else?

- If you don't like lamb, this recipe works well with beef and ground turkey.

- Harissa is a seriously fiery, highly aromatic North African spice paste with an assertive, earthy flavor. It can be hard to find (I buy it at a local Middle Eastern store, and it's available online), so if you can't get it, just use a squirt of your favorite hot sauce instead.

- Regular hamburger buns are okay to use here, though they tend to fall apart more quickly than the sturdy pita breads, especially given all the mayo you're probably going to smear on top of your burger (you'll see, it's so good you'll want more). A better, nonpita bet would be a crusty roll.

[CONTINUED]

- If you're a pickle lover (and I most definitely am), they wouldn't seem amiss here. Try stuffing a few sliced cornichons into the pita.

- Kraft mayonnaise is really better—tangier, lighter, altogether yummier—than Hellman's. In my opinion, of course.

CORN SALAD WITH TOMATOES, AVOCADOS, AND LIME CILANTRO DRESSING

Even more so than corn on the cob swabbed with butter, when summer comes, I look forward to sweet, nubby corn salads loaded with vegetables and a zesty dressing. This one is my favorite of many corn salad possibilities, mostly because of the creaminess of the avocado. It's so softly pleasant on the tongue next to all those crunchy corn kernels and juicy bits of tomato. It's a perfect party salad because you can make it ahead and it can sit out all day without wilting. But once it hits the table, I guarantee it won't last long. It's just the kind of thing that people go nuts for, no matter what else is on offer.

Serves 4 to 6

3 ears corn, kernels sliced from cob
2 tablespoons freshly squeezed lime juice
2 garlic cloves, finely chopped
1/2 teaspoon kosher salt, plus additional to taste
1/2 teaspoon freshly ground black pepper
1/4 cup extra-virgin olive oil
1 large tomato, diced
2 ripe avocados, diced
2 scallions, finely chopped
1/4 cup chopped fresh cilantro

1. Bring a medium pot of water to a boil. Drop in the corn and cook until just tender, about 2 minutes. Drain.
2. In a bowl, whisk together the lime juice, garlic, salt, and pepper. Whisk in the oil.
3. In a large bowl, combine the corn, tomato, avocados, scallions, and cilantro. Add the dressing and toss well to coat. Serve immediately.

What Else?

- If you have leftover boiled corn, you can slice off the kernels and use them for this salad, no additional boiling required. This also works with leftover grilled corn. The charred flavor is absolutely delicious.

- If it's really hot out, too hot to want to put a pot of water on to boil, I'll cook the corn on the cob in the microwave, then slice off the cooked kernels when cool. The timing will vary depending on your microwave model, but usually 4 minutes will cook 3 ears of corn. (Shuck them first.)

- A minced jalapeño or two spices things up nicely here.

A Dish by Another Name

This salad is my basic template for corn salads of every stripe. Just chop up whatever you've got that needs to get eaten and it will probably taste delicious. If you're at a loss, here are a couple of ideas:

- For Corn Salad with Red Pepper, Basil, and Olives, leave out the avocados and add 1 large diced red pepper. Substitute basil for the cilantro and lemon juice for the lime juice. Then stir in half a cup of sliced olives.

- For Corn, Tomato, and Barley Salad, omit the avocado and add 1 cup cooked barley. Season with more olive oil, salt, and lime juice to taste.

MAPLE BLUEBERRY TEA CAKE WITH MAPLE GLAZE

It takes a tremendous amount of willpower for me to bake this cake. Whenever I bring home a pint of blueberries from the market, I immediately gobble them all up, aided by Dahlia, who loves blueberries best, despite the fact that she can't stick them onto her fingers like hats, raspberry style. Leaving some for cake or crisp or anything that requires forethought seems nearly impossible when the plump, fleshy berries are in the room.

Of course I do have a few tricks I can pull out when necessary. So when I decided I wanted to make a blueberry loaf cake for midafternoon snacking, I bought an extra pint of berries and hid it in the back of the fridge behind the eggs until I was ready to bake.

By the time I pulled out the pint a few days later, it was reduced by about half (turns out Daniel especially loves blueberries in his smoothies). Luckily, there were still just enough for cake.

I added whole wheat flour to the batter of my usual buttery loaf cake recipe to give it richness and cut some of the sweetness of the cake itelf, which I intended to heap back on in the form of a maple syrup glaze. The result was a moist, fine-crumbed loaf with plenty of jammy purple pockets, well worth the delayed berry gratification to bake.

Makes 1 (8-inch) loaf cake

FOR THE CAKE

3/4 cup plus 2 tablespoons all-purpose flour

3/4 cup plus 2 tablespoons whole wheat flour

1 1/2 teaspoons baking powder

1/4 teaspoon baking soda

1/4 teaspoon kosher salt

2/3 cup pure maple syrup, preferably Grade B

1 large egg, lightly beaten

[CONTINUED]

½ cup milk

6 tablespoons (¾ stick) unsalted butter, melted

1 cup fresh blueberries

3 tablespoons maple syrup

3 tablespoons unsalted butter

Pinch kosher salt

¼ cup confectioners' sugar

1. Preheat the oven to 400°F. Lightly grease an 8-inch loaf pan.

2. In a large bowl, combine the flours, baking powder, baking soda, and salt.

3. In a separate bowl, whisk together the maple syrup, egg, milk, and melted butter. Pour the maple syrup mixture into the flour mixture and fold together until just combined. Gently fold in the blueberries. Pour the batter into the prepared pan. Bake until golden brown and a tester inserted into the middle comes out clean, 50 to 60 minutes.

4. Transfer the cake to a wire rack set over a rimmed baking sheet; cool completely. Once cool, run the tip of a knife or an offset spatula around the edges of the pan to loosen the cake. Place a plate over the pan. Flip the cake onto the plate. Tap the sides and top of the pan to help release the cake (the berries might have gotten stuck and this helps unstick them). Remove the pan. Turn the cake right-side up and put on a rack-lined baking sheet.

5. In a small saucepan over medium heat, make the glaze: Stir together the maple syrup, butter, and salt until combined. Stir in the sugar and cook until completely dissolved. Pour the warm glaze over the cake, allowing the excess glaze to drip onto the baking sheet. Slice and serve.

What Else?

- Raspberries, cubed nectarines, or peaches can stand in for the blueberries. Or use a combination of fruit if you haven't saved enough of any one.

- Try fine cornmeal in place of whole wheat flour for a sandier, coarser cake with a pretty yellow, sweet crumb.

- If you leave off the glaze, this cake becomes muffin-like and suitable for breakfast.

- I like Grade B maple syrup for baking because it has a more intense flavor than Grade A, but use what you've got. It's a pretty minor difference once it's baked into a cake.

FRESH PEACH BUTTERMILK ICE CREAM

I've always adored peach ice cream, even when I was a kid. I remember the day I discovered that Häagen-Dazs had discontinued Elberta Peach from its line. I was so upset I wrote the company a letter—a heartfelt but misspelled missive possibly penned in crayon—which yielded a nice note back and several certificates for free pints of other flavors. But alas, there was no real peachy satisfaction.

This icy memory has stayed with me. And I've spent a small chunk of my adult life churning my own peach ice cream every summer in an attempt to mimic that glorious balance of cream, egg yolk, and peaches, seasoned with just enough sugar to set off the fruit flavor without making my teeth ache.

Considering that I was barely old enough to read the ice cream label when the flavor was nixed, it's likely my childhood taste memory might be skewed to lofty levels of ice-cream perfection. And at this point, re-creating Elberta Peach is beside the point. But the tradition of making peach ice cream has stuck with me as tenaciously as the Mister Softee song, and I make it every year, adjusting the levels of sugar, lemon juice, and salt to accent the ripe peaches and cream.

Usually I stick to a very basic custard as the base, but last year I decided I wanted something a bit fresher. So I cut the cream with buttermilk. It makes a smooth, tangy ice cream that complements the peaches in a sour cream way, but lighter, brighter, and altogether more summery. It's definitely not the Elberta Peach of my childhood, but I think my adult self likes it even better.

1¹/₂ pounds fresh peaches, peeled, pitted, and diced

¹/₃ cup plus 1¹/₄ cups packed light brown sugar

Few drops freshly squeezed lemon juice

2 cups heavy cream

¹/₄ teaspoon kosher salt

Makes a
generous quart

6 large egg yolks

1½ cups buttermilk

1. In a small saucepan, combine the peaches and ⅓ cup sugar. Bring to a simmer and cook until the sugar dissolves and the fruit just begins to release its juices, 2 to 3 minutes. Stir in the lemon juice. Transfer the peaches to the blender and puree until chunky-smooth.

2. In a medium-size heavy saucepan, bring the cream, ¾ cup sugar, and salt to a simmer; turn off the heat.

3. In a large bowl, whisk the egg yolks and the remaining ½ cup sugar.

4. Remove the cream mixture from the heat and drizzle a small amount into the yolks slowly, whisking constantly to keep the eggs from curdling. Do this a few more times to warm up the yolks before pouring the yolk mixture back into the cream, whisking constantly.

5. Cook over low heat until the mixture is thick enough to coat the back of a spoon. Strain the mixture and whisk in the buttermilk. Cool completely. Freeze in an ice-cream maker according to the manufacturer's directions. When the ice cream has reached a soft-serve consistency, transfer to a bowl and swirl in the peach mixture with a quick folding action. Serve immediately.

What Else?

- Nectarines or plums can be substituted for the peaches, though you will probably want to decrease the lemon juice and increase the sugar slightly since they are tangier.

- For a more traditional ice cream, replace the buttermilk with regular milk or half-and-half.

- Try your best to serve this right out of the ice-cream maker. The silky soft-serve texture is amazing. If you have to make it ahead, let it sit out at room temperature for at least 15 minutes before serving.

[CONTINUED]

- Try topping this with caramel sauce. It's divine. Chopped pistachios are another great, colorful topping. Or use both for sweetness and crunch.

A Dish by Another Name

- For Ginger Peach Ice Cream, simmer the cream with a tablespoon of grated ginger for a few minutes. Let the cream cook, then bring to a simmer again with the sugar and proceed with the recipe, substituting regular milk for the buttermilk.

BERRY SUMMER PUDDING WITH ROSE-SCENTED CUSTARD

It wouldn't be the Fourth of July without a barbecue at my friends Karen and Dave's house, a convivial event that includes an icy bowl of strong punch, a spirited reading of the Declaration of Independence, copious amounts of grilled leg of lamb, and for dessert, Karen's opulently purple berry summer pudding, dripping with crème anglaise.

This version is pretty faithful to Karen's recipe, with two tiny tweaks: I use soft whole wheat bread in place of white bread for the pudding mold and rose water in place of lavender flowers for the creamy sauce. Since the bread is covered with all those luscious berries, you can't really tell the difference between soft whole wheat and plain white, so I figure I might as well add a few grams of fiber. And since I didn't have any lavender flowers around when I made this, I reached for the most floral substitute I could find.

It's an ideal summer dessert because you can make it ahead, it doesn't require turning on the oven, and it takes excellent advantage of all the berries of the season. And if those aren't reasons enough to make it, here is one more: It's absolutely fantastic.

Serves 8

FOR THE PUDDING

1½ pounds mixed berries (about 5 cups)

½ cup sugar, or to taste

1 to 2 teaspoons freshly squeezed lemon juice, to taste

10 to 15 slices soft whole wheat Pullman loaf, crusts removed

FOR THE CRÈME ANGLAISE (MAKES ABOUT 2½ CUPS)

1 cup whole milk

1 cup heavy cream

[CONTINUED]

6 egg yolks

1/2 cup sugar

Pinch salt

2 teaspoons rose water or vanilla extract, or to taste

1. To make the pudding, combine the berries, sugar, and 1/3 cup water in a medium saucepan. Simmer over medium heat until the sugar is completely dissolved and the berries release their juices, about 5 minutes. Stir in the lemon juice. The sauce should be sweet, with a hint of tartness. Adjust with more sugar or lemon juice as needed.

2. Spoon an even layer of berry syrup (not the berries themselves) in the bottom of an 8-inch loaf pan. Line the bottom and sides of the pan with a single layer of bread; cut the bread into pieces as necessary to fit. Spoon a third of the fruit on top of the bread, making sure the bread is completely coated; top with a layer of bread. Spoon another third of the fruit over the bread; top with another layer of bread. Spoon the remaining third of the fruit over the bread. Let the mixture cool completely, then wrap the pan tightly with plastic wrap. Place a light weight (a thick and preferably trashy paperback novel is perfect) on top of the pudding. Refrigerate overnight.

3. To make the crème anglaise, prepare a large ice water bath. Bring the milk and cream to barely a simmer in a heavy-bottomed saucepan (bubbles will just begin to form around the edges).

4. In a bowl slightly smaller than the ice water bath, whisk together the yolks, sugar, and salt. Slowly whisk in the hot milk until fully incorporated. Return the mixture to the pot. Cook, stirring constantly over medium-high heat, until the sauce is thick enough to coat the back of a spoon (170°F). Strain the sauce through a fine-mesh sieve into a metal bowl. Stir in the rose water. If it needs a bit more, go ahead and add it, but please have a light touch or it might wind up tasting like soap. Place the bowl into the water bath and stir occasionally until completely cool.

5. Run a knife around the sides of the summer pudding, then turn it over onto a plate to unmold. Serve in slices, with the custard on the side.

What Else?

• You can skip the custard sauce and serve this with whipped cream or ice cream. Since there is no butter in the pudding itself, it greatly benefits from something rich on the side.

• A mix of as many different kinds of berries as you can find is ideal. I made it with a mix of raspberries, blueberries, and blackberries, and it was lovely.

• Karen goes out of her way to use fresh currants in the berry mix. Besides adding great flavor, they also bleed lots of juice, which is what you want to help cover up all the pale bread. As she says, "It's always so sad to see the white bread peeking through." So do the same if you can find them.

• Don't try to use anything but fluffy whole wheat bread here, the soft-crusted, kid-friendly, supermarket kind and not the crusty, seed-filled, fancy-bakery/health-food-store kind. If you can't get soft whole wheat bread, use white.

A Dish by Another Name

• To make Summer Pudding with Lavender Crème Anglaise, omit the rose water and simmer the cream with a teaspoon of dried lavender for a few minutes. Let cool, then proceed with the custard recipe.

AUGUST

A PERFECT TOMATO SANDWICH

Of all the seasonal produce that I wax poetic about in these pages, nothing gives me goose bumps like a ripe summer tomato.

Meaty and succulent, its velvety flesh enclosing a fragrant jelly of golden seeds and dripping with sweet pink juice, a summer tomato is everything its cold-weather counterpart isn't, including cheap and abundant.

In August, farm stands are rich with them, laid out on tables like a re-splendent mosaic in shades of red and orange, yellow and gold, even purple, black, and green. Stunning to look at, better to eat.

And I use them in nearly everything—anything that would benefit from a sweet jolt of tomato juiciness, be it a cold, gazpacho-like soup or a warm, buttery tart.

But of all the glorious tomato possibilities, I will stand by this statement: Nothing, and I mean nothing, beats a good old tomato sandwich.

Tomato sandwiches and I go way back. I've always had a fondness for them ever since I read *Harriet the Spy* in third grade. Unlike Harriet, who likes hers on soft white bread for lunch every day, I like mine on toast to give it some crunch (and stave off the soggy factor). The toast, along with the tomatoes, is the only constant element in what is an ever-changing sandwich. I vary the fat (there has to be fat to bring out the flavor of the tomato), swap up the sea-sonings (salt, pepper, garlic, smoked paprika), and add in whatever little savory extras I've got on hand.

Given my predilection for variation, it's hard for me to pin down an exact recipe. But I'm going to try, because sometimes it's nice to have a plan before attacking a tomato in a ravenous fog. The recipe that follows makes a simple sandwich that doesn't seem like much on paper, but believe me, when made with a couple of bursting-with-juice heirloom tomatoes that have never seen a fridge, good crusty, firm bread, creamery butter that tastes like sunshine, and a generous sprinkle of crunchy sea salt, it's about the most perfect thing a person could eat on a sultry August afternoon. Or morning. Or night. A tomato sandwich is wonderful anytime—anytime in tomato season, that is.

2 slices crusty bread with a dense crumb

1 or 2 ripe tomatoes, depending upon how big the tomatoes are,
   how hungry you are, and how large your bread slices are

At least 1 tablespoon good butter

Flaky sea salt and freshly ground black pepper to taste

1. Toast the bread until crunchy and golden. While it's toasting, slice the tomatoes, taking out the brown core.

2. As soon as the toast is ready, spread it thickly with the butter. And I mean thickly, using at least a tablespoon and probably a lot more. I use about a tablespoon and a half, but then again my bread slices are on the commodious side. If the butter isn't salted, sprinkle a little salt on top, then top with the tomatoes. You can overlap them or not, depending on how thickly you've sliced them.

3. Sprinkle the tomatoes with salt and grind on some fresh black pepper. Eat with your hands. A knife and fork here diminishes the tactile pleasure.

What Else?

- Don't use ciabatta, or the tomato jelly will fall through those characteristic holes, and you want all that good stuff in your mouth.

- Other than that, you can use any bread that you like, and I've probably used every type of bread under the New York City sun, including challah (sweet and eggy), cinnamon raisin (weirdly good), seeded rye, pumpernickel, and every kind of whole grain imaginable. My favorite is a slightly sour rye loaf without seeds that I get from Balthazar Bakery.

- If there is fresh ricotta in the house, I use it in place of the butter, dolloping it on the warm bread in thick, lush spoonfuls.

[CONTINUED]

- If your tomatoes are on the flabby side flavorwise, you can add a squirt of lemon juice, but don't overdo it.

- I make a cherry tomato version of this when they are the only kind of tomatoes I have on hand. The trick is to halve them, and then place them, cut-side down, on the bread so they don't roll off.

A Dish by Another Name

- For Pan con Tomate—I wrote about this a few years ago in my *New York Times* column, and it's still a favorite: Toast the bread, then rub with a cut garlic half. Drizzle with good olive oil, rub a tomato half, cut-side down, on the toasted bread, generously squeezing the insides out as you go. Drizzle on more oil (be generous here), and pile on sliced tomatoes and a generous sprinkling of flaky sea salt. This is one to eat over the sink.

- For Tomato, Avocado, and Mayo—Toast the bread, then rub with a cut garlic half. Spread with mayonnaise, layer with avocado and tomato, and drizzle with lemon juice and good salt and lots of black pepper. Butter or olive oil can stand in for the mayo.

- For Tomato, Onion, and Butter—Toast dark, grainy bread, and spread liberally with good flavorful butter. Sprinkle with salt and pepper. Layer with tomato and thinly sliced sweet onion or slivers of scallion. Decorate with chives if you have them.

- For Tomato, Anchovy, and Olive Oil—Add anchovy fillets to the Pan con Tomate.

- For Tomato, Prosciutto, and Butter—Toast a halved baguette. Spread thickly with butter, then add tomatoes, salt, pepper, prosciutto, and basil.

CREAMED, CARAMELIZED CORN

Sweet summer corn doesn't need much help. You don't even need to cook it. Dahlia loves chomping on the raw kernels straight off the just-husked cobs. But if you do want to apply heat, you can't get a recipe much easier than this caramelized creamed corn. It's become a staple in our house. It's a snap to make, it's one of the select few foods Dahlia will reliably eat, and, oh, yeah, I love it, too.

The dish doesn't actually need a recipe, though I've written one below just in case you're nervous when it comes to improvisation. But here's what I do: Slice the kernels off the corncob and measure the volume. Then measure out half as much heavy cream (or a little less). Put the corn and cream in a thick, medium-size saucepan over medium heat. Now, go do something else in the kitchen (maybe wash greens for tonight's salad) and forget about the corn. I don't leave the room because I'm liable to burn the house down if I do, but if you are more with it, you can check your e-mail or whatnot for five minutes.

Soon you'll smell something toasty and buttery and extremely tempting—that'll be the cream caramelizing in the pan. Go back to the stove. The liquid should be mostly gone and the corn should be tender. You'll notice a brown ring around the sides of the pan; that's the good stuff. Stir it into the corn. Notice that I don't use salt, herbs, or spices. You can add them if you want, but I like this as is, pure and naked and very, very corny.

And that's all there is to it! Small children will devour this. And their parents will, too.

4 ears corn, husked
3/4 cup heavy cream

1. Stand an ear of corn up on a cutting board and use a small sharp knife to slice off all the kernels.
2. Put the kernels in a heavy pot and add the cream. Bring to a simmer and let cook for about 5 minutes, until the cream around the edges of the pan turns brown and the kernels are tender. Stir the corn well, making sure to scrape the caramelized cream off the sides and bottom of the pan. Let cool for a few minutes before serving.

What Else?

• You can add all sorts of adult additions to this basic recipe. I did a blue cheese version for my *New York Times* column, adding a bit of the crumbled cheese and piling the whole thing onto sliced tomatoes. Julienned soft herbs such as basil, chives, or dill would add their green flavor and color in a happy way. And for a carbfest, you could toss this with whole wheat couscous or bow ties. Or if you want to add protein and pinkness, toss in some shrimp.

• I have made this for Daniel, who doesn't eat cream, with coconut milk. It's good but doesn't get quite as thick. However, the sweet coconut flavor is lovely and unusual. If you want a crunchy garnish, make the toasted coconut–mustard seed topping from the braised lentils on page 275 and sprinkle it over the corn. It sends this dish over the top.

• Black pepper is quite nice here, as is a pinch of chili powder if you like it spicy. It makes it less kid-friendly but spunkier.

THAI-STYLE GROUND TURKEY
WITH CHILES AND BASIL

I have a hard time categorizing this savory, zesty, garlicky dish. It's a bit like a sloppy joe, without the tomatoes or bread, or maybe vaguely like an aromatic, beanless, thinner-sauced turkey chili. It's as quick to make as a stir-fry and employs the same technique, but I don't usually associate stir-fries with nubby ground meat.

Call it what you will, it's one of my favorite easy dinners to throw together when I'm in the mood for a punchy, Thai-inflected meal but want something more wholesome and homemade than takeout.

And it really is easy, which is what you want when August's heat has rendered you unable to do much other than sit languorously in front of the computer. The hardest thing about this dish is assembling the ingredients—not that they are difficult to find apart from the fish sauce—it's just that there are a lot of them. But once you've got everything lined up on the counter, your dinner will come together in minutes, without having the stove on very long when the last thing you want is to heat up the kitchen even more than Mother Nature (or is it the god of climate change?) has seen fit to do for you.

Of course, even if you made this in the winter, its flavors would be utterly mouthwatering. It's a crave-able mix of fragrant lime, funky fish sauce, and plenty of ginger and garlic that livens up the blank canvas that is ground turkey in an entirely new way.

Serves 4

1 tablespoon soy sauce

About 1 tablespoon Asian fish sauce such as nam pla or nuoc mam,
     or to taste (see What Else? on page 237)

1/4 teaspoon finely grated lime zest

[CONTINUED]

1 teaspoon freshly squeezed lime juice

½ teaspoon sugar

1 tablespoon peanut oil

1 tablespoon finely chopped gingerroot

3 garlic cloves, finely chopped

1 jalapeño, seeded, and finely chopped

1 fat scallion, white and light green parts finely chopped,
　　greens reserved for garnish

1 pound ground turkey

½ cup chopped fresh Thai or regular basil

Coconut or regular rice, for serving (page 49, and don't use the peas)

Lime wedges, for serving

1. In a small bowl, whisk together the soy sauce, fish sauce, lime zest, lime juice, and sugar. (If you think your fish sauce is very salty, start with 2 teaspoons; you can add more at the end if the dish needs it.)

2. Heat the oil in a large skillet over medium-high heat. Add the ginger, garlic, jalapeño, and chopped scallion. Cook, stirring, until slightly softened, about a minute. Stir in the turkey. Cook the meat, breaking it up with a fork, until it is no longer pink, 5 to 7 minutes.

3. Stir in the soy sauce mixture and cook for a minute or so, until the flavors come together. Remove from the heat and stir in the basil. Scatter with the sliced scallion greens. Serve, over warm coconut or regular rice, with lime wedges on the side.

What Else?

- You are not looking for the meat to brown in this dish, so don't be disappointed when it doesn't. As soon as it loses its pink and cooks through, add the sauce to the pan. You won't miss the caramelized flavors of browning meat, because the sauce is so intense. And the turkey stays more tender without hard little brown bits to get in the way.

- I've made this same dish with ground chicken and it's not quite as good—a bit blander and softer than the turkey, and somehow more muted in terms of the intensity of the seasonings.

- If you can get dark meat ground turkey, the dish will be more flavorful still.

- I also love this with ground pork, which makes it richer and brawnier. Or use a combination of pork and turkey.

- If you see nice-looking snow peas, steam them and toss them with sesame oil and soy sauce and serve alongside. Their crisp-juicy texture and sweet flavor is very nice with the assertive flavors of the dish.

SOUTHEAST ASIAN TOMATO SALAD

I tossed this together one night to serve with the Thai-style ground turkey dish. It's a departure from my usual tomato salad, which is comprised of little more than carved-up tomatoes, torn basil, salt, and olive oil. Daniel and I eat this simple salad almost every night in tomato season, since it takes about twenty seconds to assemble and has a juicy purity of tomato flavor that I can't seem to get enough of this time of year.

But with the fish sauce, limes, scallions, and jalapeños for the turkey already sitting out within arm's reach, I decided to try something new.

It turned out to be insanely good, very tangy and a nice break from the more everyday, if tasty, tomato salads I usually make. I've since added it to our summer tomato rotation and find myself whipping it up even if I have to hunt in the cupboard for the fish sauce and sort through the vegetable bin for a jalapeño. It's worth the chase every time.

About 2 teaspoons Asian fish sauce such as nam pla
    or nuoc mam, or to taste
2 teaspoons freshly squeezed lime juice
1 teaspoon light brown sugar
2 scallions, finely chopped
1 fat garlic clove, minced (or use 2 small ones)
1/2 jalapeño, seeded, if desired, and finely chopped
3 large or 4 medium tomatoes, sliced 1/4 inch thick
2 tablespoons chopped fresh Thai or regular basil
2 tablespoons chopped fresh cilantro

Serves 4

1. In a small bowl, whisk together the fish sauce, lime juice, sugar, scallions, garlic, and jalapeño. (If you think your fish sauce is very salty, start with 1 teaspoon; you can add more at the end.)

2. Arrange the tomato slices on a plate. Spoon the dressing over the tomatoes. Let stand 10 minutes to allow the tomatoes time to release their juices. Sprinkle with basil and cilantro; serve.

What Else?

- Cucumbers, that's what else. This salad is even better with some sliced cucumbers added to the mix. I didn't have any when I first made this, but if I had, I would have replaced one of the tomatoes with a nice big Kirby cucumber, sliced thin.

- If you have access to a tender lemongrass stalk, use it here in place of the scallion or alongside it.

- Different brands of fish sauce (otherwise known as nam pla or nuoc mam) have different degrees of saltiness. It's less apparent when used in cooking, but when drizzled raw on salads you need to be careful. Start with a little and add more as you go. I used 2 teaspoons, but trust your own palate.

- If you'd rather go for a bare-bones tomato salad, leave out all the ingredients except the tomatoes, salt, and basil. Add pepper to taste and toss well with a few drops of good olive oil. That's all you need.

A Dish by Another Name

- For a Southeast Asian Tomato Noodle Salad double all the ingredients except for the tomatoes, which you should dice instead of slice. Toss with about 6 ounces of cooked rice noodles, then adjust the seasonings to taste. It will probably need a bit more fish sauce, lime juice, and sugar.

SAUTÉED SCALLOPS WITH TOMATOES AND PRESERVED LEMON

For years, Daniel and I harbored a small jar with one homemade preserved lemon bobbing along in it. Because Daniel had made it himself, the last of a long-ago, bachelor-days batch, we neither had the heart to eat it (it was the *last* one) nor throw it out. So it sat there for years, a floating, sunny presence next to the pepper jelly, miso, lard, and other back-of-the-fridge ephemera.

Of course the minute after I finally did toss it out in a flurry of obsessive fridge cleaning, I regretted it. Preserved lemons, if you actually use them, can be a culinary treasure. They are one of those secret seasonings that makes everything you use them in taste better—brighter, more intense, and more aromatic.

From then on, I vowed to always keep preserved lemons on hand and to cook with them often.

So I bought a small jar from a nearby specialty shop. Then, as soon as I got home, I immediately pureed those cute, whole little lemons (taking out the seeds first) in the food processor and covered them with a bit of olive oil. That way whenever I wanted a little of that musky, zesty, earthy complexity that preserved lemons bring, I could just spoon some out and drop it into the pan or bowl or plate without having to stop and chop (though you could mince it up as needed if you like).

In this buoyant, tangy scallop dish, I added a dollop of the salty yellow paste to a pan of buttery scallops and chopped juicy tomato. The lemon brightened the flavors and added that extra-special layer of exotic flavor that plain citrus fruit just doesn't have. And the recipe was about as simple as can be—instant gratification that took several years to puzzle out.

1½ tablespoons unsalted butter
2 garlic cloves, finely chopped
1 pound sea scallops, patted dry
1 medium tomato, cored and chopped
1 tablespoon finely chopped or pureed preserved lemon
Kosher salt and freshly ground black pepper to taste

Melt the butter in a large skillet over medium heat. Add the garlic and cook, stirring, until fragrant, about 1 minute. Add the scallops, tomato, lemon, and a pinch of salt. Cook, stirring, until the scallops are just opaque, about 2 minutes. Season with additional salt, if needed, and pepper.

What Else?

- If you don't have preserved lemon, don't bother making this recipe. There is nothing that I can think of that can substitute for its funky, salty, citrus flavor in such a minimalist setting as this. If you have scallops, you could try the olive variation that follows, but it will be a whole new dish—still delicious, but completely different.

- Shrimp can stand in for the scallops. So can bay scallops, but you won't need to cook them as long.

- An herb is nice here and would add color. Chopped chives, chervil, basil, or mint can be stirred in at the very end just before serving.

- I like to serve this with noodles or couscous to soak up the buttery sauce.

A Dish by Another Name

- For Scallops with Olives, Tomato, and Lemon substitute a tablespoon of minced green olives mixed with an anchovy and some grated lemon zest. You'll get a tangy, complex, wonderful dish with a similar depth to the lemony original, with ingredients you probably have in the fridge.

GRILLED CUMIN AND CHILE VEAL MEATBALLS

There are a lot of people who won't eat veal on moral grounds, with good reason. Mass-produced veal raising is notoriously cruel, with calves tethered in tiny pens and fed a diet of skim milk formula to produce white-fleshed, anemic animals, who are then given a steady cocktail of hormones, steroids, and antibiotics. To add insult to injury, that kind of veal just doesn't even taste very good. It's tender, sure, but bland.

Happily these days you also have the choice of purchasing veal that both tastes delicious (sweet and delicately beefy) and is humanely raised (not surprisingly, the two go hand in hand). And I encourage all carnivores to seek out quality veal and make it a regular part of your dinner repertoire.

Why? The reason is this: Assuming you consume dairy, and assuming you purchase said dairy products from a reputable local farm that abides by sustainable raising practices, then you should know that they probably have an excess of baby bull calves cavorting around their pastures. For a cow to continue lactating, she must produce offspring. Some of that offspring will inevitably be male. Financially there is little incentive for farms to raise bull calves if no one is buying veal, which leaves them little choice but to sell them to larger producers enmeshed in the dreaded CAFO system (Concentrated Animal Feeding Operations, also known as factory farms).

On the other hand, if there's a market for humanely raised veal (like your family, for example), the male offspring can be raised responsibly and then sold at your local farm stand. It's a win-win situation for everyone. You support the farmer's livelihood, the calf gets to continue cavorting in pastureland (for a little while, anyway), and you get a tasty dinner.

For example, these veal meatballs. They are lighter and sweeter than beef meatballs, and deeply aromatic, too, because the mild veal absorbs the flavors of cumin and chile really well. I'll often make a double batch and store the

[CONTINUED]

uncooked meatballs in the freezer. They thaw in about an hour on the counter, and I can broil or grill them up whenever a meatball mood descends.

1 teaspoon whole cumin seed
1/4 teaspoon red chile flakes
1 pound ground veal
1/3 cup bread crumbs
1/4 cup chopped fresh mint or basil
1 large egg
1 garlic clove, minced
1/2 teaspoon kosher salt
1/4 teaspoon freshly ground black pepper
Olive oil, for brushing

Makes about
16 meatballs

Serves 4

1. In a dry skillet over medium heat, toast the cumin seed until fragrant, about 2 minutes. Add the chile flakes and toast 30 seconds longer.
2. In a large bowl, combine the veal, bread crumbs, mint or basil, egg, garlic, salt, pepper, and toasted spices. Mix until just combined. Form into 1-inch meatballs; thread them onto metal skewers. Brush the meatballs lightly with oil.
3. Preheat the grill to high heat and lightly brush the grate with oil. Place the skewers on the grill. Close the cover and cook, turning once halfway through, until the meatballs are golden and just firm, 5 to 7 minutes total.

What Else?

- I like the crunch and burst of flavor that you get from biting into a whole cumin seed, which is why I've used them here (and all over this book). But if you don't appreciate these qualities, you can use mellower ground cumin instead.

- Lamb is a great substitute for veal, and will give you a more flavorful, gamier meatball. Pork and turkey work, too.

- I've made these in the broiler, too. Just spread them out on a baking sheet and broil on high, as close to the broiler unit as you can get. They will take about 5 or 6 minutes. Make sure to turn them once.

- Grated orange or lemon zest makes these a bit brighter tasting, so sometimes I add a pinch. But usually I don't bother since they are so good without it.

- If you like using bamboo skewers on the grill, I won't stop you. But I hate them. No matter how long I soak them (even overnight), they always char and burn and often catch fire. I swear by my metal skewers.

- To make spaghetti and meatballs, you can brown the meatballs in a pan, then add some of your favorite tomato sauce (or use the recipe on page 325). Simmer until the meatballs are cooked through, then serve over pasta with lots of grated cheese if everyone in your house can eat it.

- You can probably get humanely raised, pastured veal at your local farmers' market. The meat will have a pink rather than white color. So-called rose veal will be somewhat less tender because all that running around outside develops muscle tone, but the mineral, delicate flavor more than makes up for it.

  If you are shopping at the supermarket, you might get lucky and find rose veal. It is sometimes sold under the following names: meadow, red, rose, pastured, grass-fed, free-range, and suckled. You can also look for the Certified Humane label (awarded by the Humane Farm Animal Care, a Humane Society and ASPCA-approved organization). This label guarantees that dairy beef calves have been raised confinement-free, with a diet that satisfies their nutritional needs, including iron and fiber.

SHAVED ZUCCHINI AND AVOCADO SALAD WITH GREEN GODDESS DRESSING

I was a green goddess once, sort of. It was in high school, where I had a very brief solo in the school play. I cannot for the life of me remember what that play was, but my part involved me singing a little song while wearing a sea green toga and gold slippers in the latest goddess fashion.

If it weren't for the fact that I happen to love the creamy, anchovy saltiness of green goddess salad dressing, I probably wouldn't have even remembered this fifteen seconds of teenage fame. But now every time I whip up a batch of the herb-flecked emulsion, my mind flits over to those bright lights, briefly cringing at the memory before concentrating on the yumminess in front of me.

And this green goddess dressing is extremely good, a classic that I don't muck with very much. I've just tweaked the herb varieties and quantities to my liking, combining a lot of pungent parsley with a bit of cilantro and a touch of basil. I also use buttermilk as the base, which gives the dressing a lighter texture compared to the sour cream and mayonnaise-laden versions you often see.

Green goddess dressing tastes good on almost any kind of vegetable matter (and fish, too); here I drizzle it all over thinly sliced rounds of zucchini and chunks of velvety avocado. It's the sort of thing I'll make when it's so hot out that all of the greens in the farmers' market look wilted and sad, but the zucchini are small, taut, and shining, just waiting to be lunch.

FOR THE GREEN GODDESS DRESSING

Serves 4

1/2 cup packed plus 2 tablespoons basil leaves

1/2 cup buttermilk

1/3 cup packed parsley leaves

1/4 cup packed cilantro leaves

3 tablespoons olive oil

2 scallions, white and light green parts, sliced

1 anchovy fillet
1 small garlic clove, finely chopped
2$\frac{1}{2}$ teaspoons freshly squeezed lemon juice
$\frac{1}{4}$ teaspoon kosher salt, plus additional to taste
Freshly ground black pepper to taste

1 medium zucchini or summer squash (about 8 ounces)
1 avocado, peeled, pitted, and cut into chunks

1. Combine the dressing ingredients in a blender and puree until smooth.
2. Using a mandoline or a very sharp knife, thinly slice the zucchini into rounds. Combine in a bowl with the avocado.
3. Pour enough dressing over the squash and avocado mixture to lightly coat the salad. Reserve any remaining dressing for another use. Serve immediately.

What Else?

- Make sure to buy small, tender, thin-skinned zucchini, which have a nice sweet flavor without any trace of bitterness. Big old leathery ones just won't do.

- This dressing is good on anything, and I mean anything: Watercress, arugula, romaine lettuce, sliced radishes, and even poached salmon will all happily sport it.

- If you want to turn this into a dip, substitute sour cream or mayonnaise or a combination for the buttermilk. I especially like serving it with whole wheat crackers and carrots. Dahlia likes it like that, too.

- Another pretty salad is made by grating some nice fresh carrots and tossing the green goddess dressing with the orange shreds. The sweetness of the carrots works really well with all the tangy herbs.

SEARED MACKEREL WITH SMOKY PAPRIKA AND SWEET PEPPERS

Some people think mackerel is a fishy fish and avoid it. I have to admit that for years I was one of them. I assumed that any fish I saw more often listed on the labels of cat food cans than on restaurant menus must be . . . let's say, strong.

But you know what? I was wrong. Fresh mackerel is sweet and buttery, with soft flaky flesh and a clean, ocean-like flavor. Moreover, it's sustainable, cheap, and healthful (high in omega-3s), all of which made me finally pick up a piece at the farmers' market a few years ago.

Well, it was all of those factors combined with the urgings of the fishmonger, who had also turned me onto porgy, another wonderful, inexpensive, sustainable sea creature that I'd ignored for too long.

He promised me that if I took care not to overcook the mackerel and served it with a drizzle of lemon or vinegar to offset the richness, I'd be rewarded with one of the finest fish dinners for two I could get for under $10.

He was right, and I've cooked up mackerel regularly ever since. Usually I keep it fairly simple, just give it a sear in olive oil and finish with a squeeze of lemon and some flaky salt. But when I want something more festive, I'll throw some onions and peppers in the pan, which accentuate the fish's natural sweetness and add color besides. It's a terrific dish that Daniel and I love to eat. Emma, our cat, however, has not been at all interested.

Serves 4

1¼ pounds mackerel fillets
½ teaspoon kosher salt, more for seasoning
½ teaspoon freshly ground black pepper, more for seasoning
½ teaspoon smoked sweet paprika
6 tablespoons extra-virgin olive oil, more as needed
2 leeks, white and light green parts only, thinly sliced

1 small red bell pepper, thinly sliced
1 small orange or yellow bell pepper, thinly sliced
5 large marjoram or thyme sprigs
3 garlic cloves, minced
⅓ cup not-too-dry white wine
Fresh lemon juice to taste
Lemon wedges, for serving

1. Season the mackerel with salt, pepper, and paprika. Let the fillets rest at room temperature while preparing the vegetables.

2. Set a large skillet over medium heat and add 5 tablespoons oil. Add the leeks, sweet peppers, marjoram, and a large pinch of salt and pepper. Cook the vegetables until they soften, about 10 minutes. Add the garlic, stirring gently, and cook for 2 minutes more. Add the wine and cook until most of the liquid has evaporated, about 5 minutes. Season to taste with more salt, pepper, and lemon juice, then transfer to one side of a serving platter.

3. Wipe the skillet with a paper towel, add the remaining tablespoon oil, and set over high heat. When the oil is hot, add the mackerel in one layer, skin-side down. Cook for 3 minutes, then flip and cook for 1 to 2 minutes longer, until the fish is cooked through. Add the fillets to the platter and spoon the vegetables on top of the fish. Serve with lemon wedges.

What Else?

- Arctic char, wild salmon, and trout are good mackerel substitutes if you really don't like mackerel. Porgy works, too, and only needs 2 or 3 minutes of cooking time total.

- Don't buy king mackerel if you see it. Because it's such a large fish, it tends to be high in mercury. Try to get the smaller Boston (Atlantic) or Spanish mackerel instead.

[CONTINUED]

- I've made this with rosé wine and it was delicious. I imagine a fruity light red would work, too, if you've got that open. Or try dry vermouth.

- For a basic version of this that doesn't require chopping any vegetables, you can skip the entirety of step 2. Just season the mackerel, let it rest for about 10 minutes, then sauté in oil as directed in step 3. Put it on top of a nice pile of bitter greens tossed with olive oil and plenty of lemon juice, and dinner is served.

ISRAELI COUSCOUS WITH FRESH CORN, TOMATOES, AND FETA

Whole wheat Israeli couscous is technically pasta—semolina flour and water rolled into little pasta balls. (Regular couscous is even tinier pasta balls, by the way.) But whenever I contemplate what to do with it, I consider it a grain—a fast-cooking, nubby little grain that's as fat and round as barley (though less starchy) and as earthy tasting as farro (though less chewy).

Usually, I just serve it as a side dish for saucy sautés, the kind with lots of pan juices for the couscous to absorb. But I also like it in this colorful summery dish, which is a cross between a warm salad and a pilaf. Folding the corn and tomato into the couscous while it is still warm brings out the vegetables' flavor, softening them slightly and making them even juicier than they started out. It also makes the feta cheese very creamy.

If you do have leftovers, it will make a marvelous light lunch the next day, though you might want to pop the couscous into the microwave for just a few seconds to make everything nice and supple, especially if you've stored it in the fridge.

Serves 6

1 large garlic clove, minced

$3/4$ teaspoon plus 1 pinch kosher salt, or to taste

2 teaspoons freshly squeezed lemon juice

$1/4$ teaspoon freshly ground black pepper

3 tablespoons extra-virgin olive oil

$1 1/2$ cups Israeli couscous, preferably whole wheat

1 cup fresh corn kernels (from 1 large ear)

1 large ripe tomato, diced

3 ounces crumbled feta cheese (optional)

2 tablespoons chopped fresh basil

[CONTINUED]

1. Using a mortar and pestle or the flat side of a knife, mash the garlic and a pinch of salt to a paste. In a small bowl, whisk together the garlic paste, lemon juice, remaining 3/4 teaspoon salt, and pepper. Whisk in the olive oil.
2. Cook the couscous according to package instructions; add the corn for the last 5 minutes of cooking. Drain well.
3. In a large bowl, combine the hot couscous-corn mixture, tomato, and vinaigrette. Let the couscous cool for about 10 minutes before gently folding in the feta, if using, and basil.

What Else?

Just about anything goes with this terrific little dish and you can vary the vegetables, herbs, and cheese to match your mood and what's in season. Here are just a few ideas:

- Chopped spinach will wilt appealingly if you fold some into the hot couscous, sautéed mushrooms make it autumnal, and roasted red peppers are an excellent substitute for the tomato.

- Parmesan cheese will give the dish added depth of flavor, and ricotta salata is just tasty anywhere you use it.

- Fresh rosemary is very appealing to use here in place of the basil for several reasons. It's less likely to turn black when you toss it with the warm couscous and therefore makes a better presentation. And I love its piney scent with fresh summer tomatoes and briny feta.

- The textural aspect of the juicy bursting nibs of corn really is nice. I would say it might be even worth using good frozen corn if you can't get good sweet fresh corn. But that depends entirely upon how you feel about frozen corn.

UPSIDE-DOWN POLENTA PLUM CAKE

There is cake served with fruit compote, and then there is an upside-down cake. The two are similar on the surface—both consist of cakes topped with cooked sugared fruit—but the differences in texture and flavor are profound. Upside-down cake is better.

This is because spreading a layer of sweetened fruit beneath the batter accomplishes several delectable things. The compote continues to caramelize in the oven, turning butterscotchy, candied, and shiny, while delicately flavoring the cake batter through and through. Plus, in this particular example, the syrupy topping helps keep the cake moist for several days, while the cornmeal in the batter keeps everything from getting soggy.

I make a version of this rustic, coarse-crumbed upside-down cake all year long, varying the fruit to match what's around. But summer, when I always buy too much fruit to eat between market visits, is the ideal time. It's one of the few homey, not-too-sweet summer treats worth turning the oven on for. Even in August.

Serves 8

1¾ pounds plums, rinsed, pitted, and sliced ½ inch thick

1½ cups plus 2 tablespoons sugar

¾ teaspoon kosher salt

1 cup fine cornmeal

½ cup all-purpose flour

1½ teaspoons baking powder

1 cup (2 sticks) unsalted butter, at room temperature

4 large eggs

⅓ cup sour cream or plain whole milk yogurt

2 teaspoons vanilla extract

Whipped cream or ice cream, for serving (optional)

[CONTINUED]

1. Preheat the oven to 350°F. Line a 9-inch springform pan with parchment paper and grease the parchment and pan well.

2. In a large skillet over medium-high heat, cook the plums, 1/2 cup plus 2 tablespoons sugar, and 1/4 teaspoon salt, stirring occasionally, until the plums are tender and the liquid begins to reduce, about 20 minutes. Spread the mixture into the prepared pan.

3. In a bowl, whisk together the cornmeal, flour, baking powder, and remaining 1/2 teaspoon salt.

4. In the bowl of an electric mixer, cream the butter and the remaining 1 cup sugar until light and fluffy. Add the eggs one at a time and beat to combine. Beat in the sour cream and vanilla.

5. Use a spatula to fold in the dry ingredients. Scrape the batter on top of the plums and smooth with a spatula. Bake until the cake is golden and springs back when touched lightly, 45 to 55 minutes.

6. Allow the cake to cool in the pan for 10 minutes, then unmold the sides and invert onto a plate. Serve warm with whipped cream or ice cream, if desired.

What Else?

- If you don't feel like simmering up the plum compote, you can use any kind of jam in the bottom of the pan. You'll need about 1 1/2 cups. Orange marmalade is especially good because it's nice and tart. And I like it.

- You can simmer a cinnamon stick along with the plums; it will add a subtle layer of toasty spice to the juicy plums.

- Although you can probably use almost any fruit in this recipe, I like tangier, more acidic fruits best to counter all the sugar you need to use to create a caramelized topping. I think plums, rhubarb, raspberries, blackberries, cranberries, apricots, and the classic pineapple work better than milder blueberries, peaches, and pears. If you would like to use low-acid fruit, add a healthy squeeze of lemon or lime to the compote, along with grated zest if you like the flavor of it. Blueberry upside-down cake is terrific with a good jolt of lime juice and zest.

- Speaking of citrus zest, a little tangerine or lemon zest is a zippy addition in the cake batter. Or for something fragrant, try a pinch of freshly grated nutmeg or ground cardamom, which is particularly lovely with plums.

A Dish by Another Name

- For Upside-Down Fresh Pineapple-Polenta Cake, substitute 3 cups sliced fresh ($1/_2$-inch pieces) pineapple for the plums and $1/_3$ cup dark brown sugar for the granulated sugar. Cook for about 8 minutes, until tender and browned. If you want the topping to be browned and toffee-like, as you'd find on a traditional upside-down cake of the canned pineapple persuasion, add 2 tablespoons of butter to the pan when you make the compote.

- Also if you like, you can substitute 3 tablespoons maraschino liqueur for the vanilla extract in the cake (a nod to maraschino cherries in those canned pineapple upside-down cakes).

SEPTEMBER

STUPENDOUS HUMMUS

I'd never thought too hard about the divide between the pretty good hummus I'd throw together in the food processor from canned chickpeas and the extraordinary hummus I ate at certain Middle Eastern restaurants around town. My hummus was certainly tasty—garlic laden, lemony, and mixed with good, peppery olive oil and dashes of cumin and cayenne. It didn't have that satiny smooth texture or deep earthy je ne sais quoi of restaurant hummus, but it came together in minutes with a minimum of fuss, and for years that was good enough for me.

Then I made the mistake of trying out a hummus recipe from Mitchell Davis's wonderful book, *Kitchen Sense* (Clarkson Potter, 2006). I'm friendly with Mitchell (a muckety-muck at the James Beard Foundation and a well-known figure on the New York City food scene) and have even been a dinner guest at his house. He's a terrific cook who knows his stuff. So when he proclaimed a hummus recipe the best you've ever tasted, well, I had to try it.

The first thing that makes Mitchell's recipe different from most is that not only does he insist upon using freshly cooked chickpeas instead of canned, he also strongly implores you to peel the peas.

Yup, you read that right. Peel the chickpeas—each, individual, tiny little pea.

I knew that was never going to happen in my kitchen. But cooking the peas from scratch? Now, that I could handle, considering all it involved was putting a pot of water and chickpeas on the fire and letting it do its thing while I did mine.

So I tried it, cooking up the peas, and pureeing them with the usual cumin-garlic-tahini-lemon mixture.

Mitchell was right. It really was by leaps and bounds the best hummus I'd ever made, with a rich, almost toasty flavor from the freshly cooked garbanzos that enhanced the fragrance of the spices, which I also sprinkled on top as a potent garnish. Maybe it wasn't quite the best I'd ever had, but considering I didn't peel the peas, I wasn't expecting that absolute hummus euphoria.

Ever since then, I only use canned chickpeas in a last-minute hummus emergency. (This happens more often than you'd think; Dahlia loves hummus, and sometimes it is all I can think of to feed her for lunch.) Otherwise, I boil up my peas to whip up a streamlined version of Mitchell's carefully wrought masterpiece.

By the way, just for comparison's sake, I did make a batch of hummus with peeled chickpeas. I rounded up a friend and we boiled a cup of chickpeas. It took the two of us working together about half an hour to slip off all the papery peels. And yes, that peel-less hummus was even better than this one—smoother, silkier, altogether more luscious. But I doubt I'll ever try that again.

Makes about 3¹/₂ cups

Freshly squeezed juice of 1 lemon, plus additional for serving

1 teaspoon kosher salt

¹/₂ teaspoon ground cumin

¹/₂ teaspoon freshly ground black pepper

1 fat garlic clove or 2 smaller cloves, finely chopped

Pinch cayenne, plus additional for serving

¹/₃ cup tahini

3 cups cooked chickpeas, preferably cooked up from dried peas (see What Else?)

¹/₂ cup extra-virgin olive oil, plus additional for drizzling

Cumin salt (see page 198) or flaky sea salt, for serving

1. Combine the lemon juice, salt, cumin, black pepper, garlic, and cayenne in a food processor. Pulse the mixture a few times until the liquid whirls around just enough to blend together. Drop in the tahini and ¹/₂ cup water. Pulse until smooth. Add the chickpeas and puree until smooth and creamy. This might take several minutes, but stick with it. With the motor running, drizzle in the oil until the mixture is combined. Taste and adjust the flavors if you think it needs it; you might need to add a pinch of salt. I used 1¹/₄ teaspoons, but it teetered on that edge of perfectly salted and too salty, so I cut it back in the ingredients list. If you do add salt, dissolve it first in a few drops of lemon juice or warm water (see What Else? for why).

[CONTINUED]

2. Spread the hummus on a plate. Top it with a generous drizzle of olive oil, a squeeze of lemon juice, and a dash of cayenne. Finish with a sprinkling of cumin salt or sea salt, and serve.

What Else?

- Combining the lemon juice with the salt and spices before adding other ingredients is a trick I learned from my friend, chef and food writer Peter Berley. The idea is that the lemon juice dissolves the salt and intensifies the spices, which helps the flavors distribute more evenly throughout the hummus.

- If you want to add more salt to your hummus after all the ingredients have been pureed, you need to dissolve it in a little water or lemon juice first. Otherwise it will be hard to get it to dissolve in the oily mixture, and you might end up oversalting by mistake.

- Yes, you can use canned, drained chickpeas in this recipe, and your hummus will be fine. But it won't be stupendous. There really is a tremendous difference in texture and flavor between canned and home cooked, and cooking the chickpeas isn't hard to do if you have the time.

- To cook your own chickpeas, soak 1 cup of them overnight in a large bowl of cold water, then simmer in a pot of heavily salted water with 4 peeled garlic cloves until tender, usually about 1 hour. (Discard the garlic.) If you don't soak them overnight, they will take 2 to 3 hours to cook, depending on the age of the beans. A cup of dried chickpeas yields 3 cups cooked.

- If you decide to cook your own chickpeas and are feeling particularly dedicated to your hummus-making project, then consider peeling the skin that clings loosely to the cooked legumes. This isn't at all essential and it's definitely a labor of love, but the creamiest, most genuinely mind-blowing hummus I've ever made was the result of this extra, somewhat insane step. Sometimes I'll stand over the pot and peel some of the chickpeas until I get bored. I figure it makes the texture slightly smoother.

- Honestly, when you don't have time to make your own hummus, put all your efforts into the cumin salt (page 198), which only takes only a minute or two. Sprinkle it over store-bought hummus with a nice slick of oil and squeeze of lemon. It will elevate even the most humble supermarket brand.

- I never serve my hummus in a bowl. I always spread it in a thick layer on a large plate, the way they do in Middle Eastern restaurants. That way each and every bite benefits from the delicious oil-lemon-cumin salt topping, which, besides looking beautiful, really makes the hummus taste even better.

ROASTED PEPPER AND CELERY LEAF CROSTINI

I adore roasted red peppers, but haven't made a proper batch in years. It's not that they are hard to do, just messy and time consuming. You have to blister the red peppers until the skins char black, then steam them in a bowl or bag until they cool, then slither off the ashen skins with your fingers, but *not* under running water or you will lose a lot of flavor. Inevitably, this peeling takes much longer than I think it will, plus the tarry bits of skin stick everywhere—counters, dish towels, under my fingernails. Cleanup is a pain.

But I love the rich, earthy flavor of roasted peppers, especially when they're piled high on a slice of garlic-rubbed crostini, maybe decorated with celery leaves and salty anchovies (or capers).

So for the last few red pepper seasons I've struck a compromise that suits my current, lazier cooking style much better. I roast the peppers until melting, caramelized, and jammy, but I don't peel them. They come out a little bit like a confit, with an intense red pepper taste. They are not as velvet textured and refined as proper roasted peppers, but they are so much easier that I find myself making them all the time (even on weeknights) and not just for a fancy party or special occasion. These days, easy satisfaction is where I'm at.

2 medium red bell peppers, seeded and cut into 1/4-inch strips

4 teaspoons extra-virgin olive oil, plus additional for
     drizzling the bread

1/2 teaspoon kosher salt

1/2 teaspoon smoked sweet paprika

1/4 cup chopped celery leaves

6 slices crusty bread, cut about 1/4 inch thick

1 garlic clove, halved

Anchovy fillets or drained capers, for serving (optional)

Makes 6 crostini

COOK *This* NOW

1. Preheat the oven to 375°F. In a bowl, toss the peppers with the olive oil, salt, and paprika. Spread on a large baking sheet and roast, stirring occasionally, until the peppers are very tender and jammy, 25 to 30 minutes. Let cool completely; toss the peppers with the celery leaves.

2. Preheat the broiler. Spread the bread slices out in an even layer on a baking pan and toast them until golden, 1 to 2 minutes. Immediately rub each slice with garlic and drizzle with oil.

3. To serve, mound the peppers on top of the bread slices. Garnish each crostini with either a single anchovy fillet or capers, if desired (about $\frac{1}{2}$ teaspoon per crostini).

What Else?

- I love these roasted peppers on their own as a side dish or tossed into salads, where they add a sweet, almost candied bite that offsets arugula and other bitter greens perfectly. I've also stirred them into pasta sauce, where they're a natural with tomatoes.

- Dahlia loves these when I serve them with the capers on top in place of the anchovies. Daniel and I like them with both anchovies and capers, though that's definitely lily painting if there ever was. If you don't like either capers or anchovies, you can use sliced pitted olives or chopped cornichons or other pickles. The point is to add a saline contrast to the peppers' rich sweetness. Another nonbrined way to go here is to top the crostini with slivers of salty prosciutto or sopressata.

- If I can get a variety of colored peppers, I mix and match them for the prettiest crostini. Red, orange, and yellow all work well, as long as they are fleshy and fat. Green peppers, which aren't as ripe, don't work as well here (since they don't have as high a natural sugar content, they don't caramelize as nicely).

PASTA WITH BACON, ROSEMARY, AND VERY RIPE TOMATOES

The only problem with tomato season is that I lose all self-restraint. I cannot seem to walk away from the farmers' market without buying bags and bags of the multicolored lovelies, more than I can possibly use before they start melting on the kitchen counter, collapsing into a sticky puddle under the weight of their own fragrant juice.

Because of this inclination toward tomatoey excess, I make this pasta dish regularly in summer. It's just the thing to absorb those oozing tomatoes that need to be used *right now* or, you know, never.

Daniel, Dahlia, and I don't mind eating this often; it's a bare-bones recipe that far transcends the sum of its parts. Taking about fifteen minutes to put together, it's a nuanced, herbal, porky combination that really tastes of fresh summer tomatoes.

If you don't happen to have dead-ripe tomatoes in want of a home, this recipe will work with regular tomatoes, too, though it may not be quite as juicy (you can add a little water if the ingredients start to stick).

Daniel and I once ate this with a green bean salad on the side (page 265) and another time paired it with sautéed Swiss chard. But any fresh green vegetable would be nice. Do not, however, omit an accompanying glass of rustic red wine—that's a must.

8 ounces pasta shape of choice (I often use farro spaghetti here)

3 ounces bacon, sliced into 1/2-inch pieces

1 large bushy rosemary sprig

2 garlic cloves, minced

Pinch crushed red pepper flakes

Kosher salt and freshly ground black pepper to taste

Serves 2

2 very large tomatoes (or 3 medium; a mix of yellow and red is nice),
    cored and chopped
Balsamic vinegar (optional)
Soft herbs, if you want this to look pretty

1. Cook the pasta in a large pot of heavily salted water.
2. Meanwhile, in a large skillet over medium heat, cook the bacon until brown, about 5 minutes. Transfer the bacon to a paper towel–lined plate, leaving the grease in the pan (if it looks really greasy, spoon some out; you just need a thin layer, enough to sauté the garlic without burning).
3. Add the rosemary, garlic, red pepper flakes, and salt and pepper to taste to the skillet and cook until the garlic is lightly browned, 1 to 2 minutes. Add the tomatoes and let the sauce simmer until the pasta is cooked. Season aggressively with more salt and black pepper. If it tastes flat, add a few drops of vinegar.
4. Drain the pasta and top with the sauce. Sprinkle with the bacon and herbs, if you like.

What Else?

- I use thick-cut bacon here, so 3 ounces worked out to be 3 thick slices. If you use thinner bacon, it might brown very quickly, so watch it carefully.

- Sometimes I add leeks or onions to the sauce. I sauté them in the bacon fat for a few minutes before adding the garlic and red pepper. You can also add chopped fennel, in which case save the fronds for garnish.

- Grated Pecorino Romano is really nice here but not essential.

- If you accidentally ended up with mealy summer tomatoes, fear not; this recipe is exactly where they belong. This used to happen to me all the time.

[CONTINUED]

I'd buy a bag of tomatoes in good faith at the farmers' market, expecting summery bliss. But when I'd dig in, I'd find their flesh as cottony as a supermarket tomato in winter, albeit a lot juicier. As long as the tomatoes have good flavor, the mealiness will disappear in the pan when you cook them.

And if you were wondering what causes mealiness in tomatoes, I can tell you because I found out. One reason is being refrigerated at supermarket warehouses. (Chilling tomatoes ruins their texture and flavor; don't do it at home either.) But mealiness can also strike seasonal, never-saw-the-fridge farmers' market tomatoes if they are overripe.

To tell the difference between ripe and overripe, cradle a tomato gently in your palm. Its skin should be taut rather than slack, and the tomato should feel as if its juices are about to burst out of the tight skin, like a water balloon just before it makes contact with your head. If it feels at all soft, leave it be and find another more likely candidate.

GREEN BEAN SALAD WITH WALNUTS AND WALNUT OIL

This is the kind of salad my mother always made whenever she could get tiny haricots verts—green beans as slender as dandelion stems. They reminded her of summer vacations in France, where she first tried them, and that association always made her pull out her can of fancy French walnut oil, which she'd drizzle judiciously over the beans to dress them.

My mother never added nuts to her salad, keeping it sweetly simple with a few drops of the fragrant oil, a squeeze of lemon, and maybe a shower of chopped garlic, left over from another dish (she would never chop garlic just for this salad, but if it were there anyway, she'd use it). The green beans invariably sat on the table next to a bowl of thickly cut tomatoes sprinkled with basil and olive oil, and we ate everything with our hands, sometimes combining both beans and tomatoes in one large bite while we listened to the buzzing *zap zap* of the electric mosquito fryer perched over the deck.

My take on green bean salad is a little more involved in that I mix together a dressing with shallot, tarragon, and sherry vinegar, and I add toasted walnuts to bring out the nuttiness of the oil. It's a less direct and immediate way to serve the beans, but I like the added texture and complexity of flavors. If I can't get pin-thin haricots verts, I'll still make this with regular green beans or wax beans. It's not as dainty, but just as tasty.

Serves 4

1/3 cup walnuts

3/4 pound green beans, preferably thin haricots verts, trimmed

2 teaspoons finely chopped shallot

1 1/2 teaspoons sherry vinegar

1/4 teaspoon kosher salt, plus additional to taste

[CONTINUED]

¼ teaspoon freshly ground black pepper,
   plus additional to taste
1½ tablespoons walnut oil
¾ teaspoon chopped tarragon

1. Preheat the oven to 350°F. Spread the walnuts on a baking sheet. Toast until golden, 7 to 10 minutes. Let the nuts cool, then chop them coarsely.
2. Bring a large pot of salted water to a boil. Drop in the green beans and cook until bright green and just shy of being crisp-tender, 1 to 2 minutes (this will take longer for thicker beans; keep testing them until they are just slightly underdone to your taste, then immediately take them off the heat). Drain well.
3. In a small bowl, whisk together the shallot, vinegar, salt, and pepper. Whisk in the walnut oil and tarragon.
4. In a bowl, toss together the walnuts, warm beans, and dressing. Taste and adjust the seasonings, if necessary. Serve warm or at room temperature.

What Else?

- Warm beans absorb the flavors of the dressing better than ice-cold beans, which is why I don't use an ice bath to stop their cooking. I simply take them off the heat about a minute or so before they are done to my liking. The residual heat finishes them nicely while they suck up all the seasonings.

- If you're not doing this already, be sure to store your nut oils in the fridge. They will go rancid really quickly if you don't.

- If you don't have walnut oil, use good olive oil. In this case, feel free to vary up the nuts. Slivered toasted almonds are nice with green beans, and I'm a big hazelnut fan as well. If you have hazelnut oil and hazelnuts, you could even swap those out for the walnuts and oil. I've done that many times and like it just as much as the walnut version.

- Halved cherry tomatoes are a nice and colorful addition.

- Basil, mint, or parsley can be substituted for the tarragon, although they won't have that potent green fennel flavor. You'll probably need to increase the amount you use to compensate for the diminished intensity.

FRESH CORN POLENTA
WITH ROASTED RATATOUILLE
AND RICOTTA

I vividly remember the first time I had ratatouille, and it had very little to do with the actual vegetable dish. That's because sitting across a wooden table from me while I ate it was a boy, perhaps fifteen to my thirteen, with a strong jaw, a head of tight brown curls, and not a word of English. We were in Cavaillon in France, having lunch with a family whose house we were about to inhabit for the month of August, exchanging their cute French farmhouse with our Victorian in Flatbush, Brooklyn. We planned this lunch as a way to overlap with the people who'd sleep in our beds and cuddle our kitty cats while we did the same thing *chez lui*.

Had I not been staring at the boy, with whom I never exchanged anything but tentative glances, I might have been more aware of the simple mound of eggplant, zucchini, and tomatoes on my plate, which, by the accounts of my parents and even my sister, was superb, marvelous, fantastic—the best ratatouille the Clark family had ever been served. Everyone lapped it up and my mother got the recipe, which she proceeded to make all summer long. Without the curly-haired boy to distract me, I soon realized just how good a pot of carefully stewed vegetables could be.

That ratatouille recipe was as traditional as they come. It called for sautéing all the elements individually, then combining them at the end. The idea is that by keeping the vegetables separate, you respect their different cooking times (so each one is cooked until just soft but not falling apart) and maintain their integrity of flavor.

While I applaud this technique, I admit that I no longer follow it. It's just too darn labor intensive, especially for summertime.

Instead, I roast everything in the oven all at once, which browns the vegetables and condenses their flavors, adding a caramel note that's absent in more classically stewed ratatouilles.

The downside is that roasting will heat up your kitchen more than stovetop cooking. But since you don't have to babysit each type of vegetable in the skillet at a time, you can retire to the air-conditioned living room while it does.

When the vegetables are bronzed and glistening and slack in the pan, I toss them with some sweet roasted garlic and a few drops of lemon juice if the caramelized flavors seem a bit cloying.

This roasted ratatouille needs nothing but a fork and plate to make it a completely satisfying culinary experience (even the plate is optional if you're the one holding the bowl). But something starchy—pasta, couscous, or soft polenta studded with fresh corn kernels—raises the dish to celestial heights. It's so compelling that even my toddler daughter will look away from her true love, Elmo, to really focus on a few bites when I put it in front of her—which is more than I can say for my thirteen-year-old self.

Serves 2 as a main dish, 4 as a side

2 small eggplants (about 3/4 pound), cut into 1-inch chunks

2 small zucchini (about 1/2 pound), cut into 1-inch chunks

2 small red bell peppers (about 1/2 pound), cut into 1-inch chunks

2 large rosemary branches

1/4 cup plus 1 teaspoon extra-virgin olive oil

Kosher salt, for seasoning

Freshly ground black pepper, for seasoning

1 pint cherry tomatoes

2 garlic cloves, unpeeled

Fresh lemon juice, as needed (optional)

FOR THE POLENTA

1 bay leaf

3/4 teaspoon salt

1 cup polenta or coarse cornmeal (see What Else?)

1 1/2 cups fresh corn kernels (from 2 small ears)

Fresh ricotta, for serving

Fresh torn basil leaves, for serving (optional)

[CONTINUED]

1. Preheat the oven to 400°F.
2. In a large bowl, toss the eggplants, zucchini, bell peppers, and 1 rosemary branch with 3½ tablespoons oil; season generously with salt and pepper. Spread the vegetables on a large baking sheet.
3. In a small bowl, toss the tomatoes, garlic, and remaining rosemary branch with ½ tablespoon oil; season with salt and pepper. Spread the mixture on a small baking sheet.
4. Transfer both baking sheets to the oven. Roast, stirring the vegetables occasionally, until they are tender and caramelized, about 25 minutes for the tomatoes and garlic; 30 to 35 minutes for the eggplants, zucchini, and peppers.
5. Let the vegetables cool for a few minutes. Slip the garlic from their skins and place the cloves in a small bowl. Add a pinch of salt and mash to a paste; whisk in the remaining 1 teaspoon oil. In a bowl, combine the garlic oil with the tomatoes, eggplants, zucchini, and peppers. Taste and add more salt and a few drops of lemon juice if it needs it.
6. Make the polenta: In a medium saucepan, bring 3 cups water, the bay leaf, and salt to a boil. Slowly whisk in the polenta; simmer it, stirring, until it is thick and almost tender, about 10 minutes. Stir in the corn and simmer 5 minutes more.
7. Spoon the polenta onto individual serving plates. Top with roasted vegetables and a dollop of ricotta and basil, if you like.

What Else?

- Here is a word about polenta because I love it and it makes such a soft, sweet, buttery bed for anything juicy and garlicky, such as this ratatouille. Polenta is coarsely ground cornmeal cooked until tender and creamy. You can buy a package labeled "polenta" from a fancy gourmet market, or you can buy regular coarsely ground cornmeal from the supermarket. It's basically the same thing. I like Bob's Red Mill brand, which cooks in 10 or 15 minutes using 3 parts salted water to 1 part meal (different brands cook at different rates, so make sure to follow the directions on the package and taste as you go; when it seems done, it is).

Sometimes I cook the polenta with a bay leaf to give it an earthy flavor. My friend Karen cooks her polenta in part milk for richness. I achieve a similar result by adding a large knob of butter to the pot.

You can also use instant polenta, which is finely ground and cooks in a minute or two. It doesn't have that chewy, gritty texture that I love in coarse, slow-cooking polenta, but you can get it on the table in minutes, which is perfect for days when you've forgotten all about making a side dish, and dinner is nearly ready (happens to me more often than I like to admit).

• If you don't want to make the polenta, you can serve this on pasta, rice, couscous, or quinoa. Or serve it as a side dish to any summer protein; grilled or sautéed meats, chicken, fish, tofu, or whatever you've got will be happy to share a plate with this deeply flavored vegetable stew.

A Dish by Another Name

• For Roasted Shrimp and Ratatouille, about 10 minutes before the ratatouille is done, pop a pan of large oiled and salted shrimp into the oven. You can add a little lemon zest to the shrimp if you like; it's a nice contrast to the sweetness of the dish.

BRAISED PORK RIBS WITH GREEN TOMATO, ORANGE, AND THYME

One summer, I enrolled in a pork CSA. It worked like this: I paid upfront for a share of a pig, and in exchange received a bimonthly bag of pork products fresh from a small family farm. I loved the suspense factor of never knowing what's for dinner until you open the bag. We've gotten thick-cut pork chops, ham hocks, the best mortadella I've ever had, smoked sliced ham, pig pâté, and lots and lots of bacon. Some of the stuff I've gobbled up after unwrapping it (did I mention it was the best mortadella I've ever had?). But I also got plenty of opportunities to expand my pig-cooking repertoire.

I came up with this recipe when I ripped open a package of meaty country-style ribs, a cut I wasn't terribly versed in (see What Else? for more details). The Internet said I could have grilled them slowly over indirect heat. But it also mentioned braising, easier at least for me and more in my comfort zone (braising = easy; grilling = not so easy). And since it was a chilly night— one of those late summer evenings where a cool, sweater-appropriate wind blows across the deck at sunset—I didn't mind turning on the oven.

Unlike most braises, which require browning the meat before slow cooking it, for this recipe I skipped that step. The meat is not as burnished and pretty as browned meat, and yes, I did lose a layer of caramelized flavor. But this streamlined technique meant keeping things quick and easy. I tossed everything together in fifteen minutes, then let it slowly cook while I bathed my daughter, put her to bed, and had a civilized predinner cocktail with Daniel before we sat down to the table to enjoy the feast.

In true improv fashion, I used the stuff I had around to flavor the pork. There were a couple of green tomatoes left over from a pie, a use-it-or-lose-it orange left over from . . . who remembers, some herbs from the deck, garlic, and vermouth from the stash in the fridge. I was happily surprised by the way the ingredients bonded. The green tomato and orange were a great match, and the basil and thyme added just the right, subtle herby notes to the rich, fatty pork. The flavors were so good together I filed the combination away in my brain under "pork." With months to go in my CSA, I knew there'd be many more pieces of pig heading my way. And I was ready for it.

Serves 4

8 country-style pork ribs (about 4 pounds)
3 tablespoons olive oil
3 or 4 garlic cloves, minced
Freshly squeezed juice and grated zest of 1 orange
Kosher salt and freshly ground black pepper to taste
2 large green tomatoes, diced
1/4 cup dry vermouth or white wine
6 bushy lemon or regular thyme sprigs
2 large rosemary sprigs
Orange wedges, for serving
Crusty bread, polenta, or rice, for serving

1. Smear the ribs all over with 1 tablespoon olive oil, the garlic, orange zest, and lots of salt and pepper. Place the tomatoes, orange juice, vermouth or wine, the remaining 2 tablespoons olive oil, and additional salt and pepper in a baking dish or roasting pan (I used a 9×13-inch baking pan) and toss well. Top with the pork ribs and herbs. Cover with foil. If you have time, let it marinate in the refrigerator for as long as you can stand it (I've left it for about 4 hours but it could go straight into the oven if need be or will be happy to sit overnight).
2. Preheat the oven to 300°F.
3. Bake, covered with the foil and turning the pork halfway through, until the meat is just falling-off-the-bone tender, about 3 hours. Season with additional salt and pepper to taste. Squeeze the orange wedges over the pork ribs before serving with bread, polenta, or rice.

What Else?

- Ripe red tomatoes work here, too, or those half-red, half-green ones you get at the end of the season. The only thing is that you'll need to adjust the acidity of the dish, since green tomatoes are a lot more tart than ripe ones. Just substitute lemon wedges for the orange wedges when serving and you should be fine.

- Country ribs are not really ribs, but a bone-in pork piece cut from the shoulder (aka the butt). I love their meaty flavor and the richness you get from cooking the meat together with their marrow-exuding bones. Sometimes you see boneless country-style ribs, but don't substitute those here. You want the bone for the maximum flavor. Better to use baby back or St. Louis ribs instead. The cooking times will stay the same.

274

SPICED BRAISED LENTILS
AND TOMATOES WITH
TOASTED COCONUT

Lentil stew sounds like the kind of mushy, nondescript '70s vegetarian dish that I avoid at all costs, no matter how much I adore lentils. Instead, I've always turned my lentils into brothy soups or textured salads.

Then I saw a recipe called braised lentils and got extremely excited. I love braised foods of all persuasions, so why not lentils? The recipe itself turned out to be disappointing—it read exactly like every other boring lentil stew recipe I'd ever seen.

But it gave me the idea to come up with a braised lentil dish of my own.

The thing that sets most braising recipes apart from stews is searing the ingredients in fat before adding the liquid. This adds a layer of good browned flavor to perfume the whole dish. So I decided to try it with lentils.

I started with a base of butter-sautéed scallions and garlic, adding spicy Madras curry powder and tomato paste for layers of flavor. Since I compulsively put tomatoes in everything when I can get good ripe ones, I stuck a couple of those in the pot, too.

Then while it simmered, I toasted coconut and mustard seeds until fragrant and golden to use as a piquant topping. It's a trick I picked up from my local Indian restaurant, which uses a similar mix on top of rice pilaf.

It added just the right note of crunchy complexity to the soft mound of spicy, tomatoey, buttery braised lentils, which, I'm happy to report, were absolutely nothing like stew. Or so I tell myself.

Serves 6

3 tablespoons unsalted butter
1 bunch scallions, white and light green parts, thinly sliced
2 garlic cloves, finely chopped
1 tablespoon good-quality Madras curry powder

[CONTINUED]

1 tablespoon tomato paste

2 cups green or brown lentils

3/4 pound ripe juicy tomatoes, chopped (2 medium)

1 3/4 teaspoons kosher salt, plus additional to taste

1 cup unsweetened coconut flakes

1 1/2 tablespoons black or brown mustard seeds

Salty butter, for serving

Plain whole milk yogurt, for serving (optional)

Chopped cilantro, for serving

1. Melt the unsalted butter in a large saucepan over medium-high heat. Add the scallions, garlic, and curry powder. Cook until the vegetables are golden and soft, about 4 minutes. Stir in the tomato paste and lentils and cook until slightly caramelized, 1 to 2 minutes. Add the tomatoes and 1 3/4 teaspoons salt. Add enough water to cover the mixture by 1/2 inch. Bring the liquid to a boil over high heat; reduce the heat to medium-low and simmer until the lentils are tender, 25 to 40 minutes. If the lentils begin to look dry while cooking, add more water, as needed.

2. In a small, dry skillet over medium heat, toast the coconut, mustard seeds, and a large pinch of salt until the coconut is golden, about 3 minutes.

3. To serve, spoon the lentils into individual bowls. Drop about 2 teaspoons salted butter into each dish. Top with yogurt, cilantro, and the coconut mixture.

What Else?

- Daniel happily devoured this without the yogurt, using parathas (page 278) to wipe his plate clean.

- Madras curry powder is a type of curry powder used in South India. It's hotter than the usual curry powders we get here. If you can't find it, use hot curry powder in its place or regular curry powder with a pinch of cayenne.

- The garnish of crunchy coconut and mustard seeds is amazing on salads if you have any left over. Try sprinkling them on top of leafy greens. It's also nice on rice dishes, soups, and braised greens. Once, I used a bit on top of some boiled collard greens, and it was a lovely, crunchy contrast to the soupy, silky greens.

- If you don't have mustard seeds, you can leave them out or substitute poppy seeds, which will give you a similar crunch and nutty flavor, if not the sparky bite of mustardy heat. Or, if you've got some of that Turkish or Syrian chili powder I've sweet-talked you into getting, use a sprinkle of it here for some heat.

- Don't substitute red lentils here because they will fall apart, which isn't a terrible thing necessarily; but I really like the beady lentil texture against the coconut chips.

- If you are making this in winter, you can use canned plum tomatoes. You'll need about 2 cups (drained). Or use a 15-ounce can of diced tomatoes.

BUTTERY WHOLE WHEAT PARATHA

When I moved in with the only vegetarian man I ever dated, I came armed with Madhur Jaffrey's *World of the East Vegetarian*. I was nineteen years old, and eager to be cooking anything with the man I loved, even if it involved mung beans rather than bacon. I spent long Saturday mornings sprawled on our futon, bookmarking recipes that we made together later that night.

Seth was definitely the better and more experienced cook, but I was fearless in the kitchen, not afraid of tackling complicated techniques or taking the L train into the city to seek out asafetida powder and nigella seeds.

With Madhur Jaffrey as our guide, we made our own paneer cheese, boiled down gallons of milk for homemade cardamom-flavored ice cream called kulfi, and even rolled and pleated a rather complicated-seeming Indian bread called paratha that puffed in the skillet as we fried them in butter.

We spent hours on those meals, starting at sunset and cooking through the night, eating multicourse dinners near midnight with whatever roommates or friends were around. We were always proud of our hard work and didn't mind the late hour, since we had nothing to get up for on Sunday morning other than each other.

When I moved out, I took Madhur Jaffrey with me, but didn't open the book again for years. The recipes were too long and complicated, I'd think when I spotted the spine on the shelf. And besides, now that I was back to dating meat eaters, why bother with vegetarian food?

Then recently, I got the urge to make parathas again. I had been making a lot of whole wheat pizza dough (page 182), and it reminded me how much I adored the whole wheat flatbreads of yore.

This time I looked online for recipes and found a bunch, all of which were pretty similar to that old Madhur Jaffrey recipe with one time-saving exception: Instead of pleating the dough into little pouches, they called for simple rolling and folding. (I later found out that Ms. Jaffrey uses this simplified technique in her latest book, *At Home with Madhur Jaffrey*, so I guess she got tired of all that fussy finger work, too.)

I whipped up a batch to serve with the Spiced Braised Lentils and Tomatoes with Toasted Coconut on page 275, and they didn't take that much longer to make than a pot of basmati rice pilaf.

Daniel, Dahlia, and I ate them up (in fact, that was pretty much all Dahlia ate since the lentils were a bust in her opinion). They were as buttery, flaky, and wheaty tasting as I remembered, but a lot less work, so we could eat them at sunset rather than midnight—a sad but necessary change from those free-flowing college days.

Makes 6 flatbreads

1 cup whole wheat flour, plus additional for dusting
1/2 teaspoon kosher salt, plus additional for seasoning
1/2 cup plus 2 tablespoons unsalted butter, melted
Nigella (black onion) seeds (optional)

1. In a large bowl, whisk together the flour and salt. Pour 4 tablespoons melted butter over the flour mixture. Use your fingers to rub the butter into the flour until the mixture becomes moist and crumbly. Knead in 1/2 cup water, a little at a time, as needed, until a soft dough forms.
2. Transfer the dough to a lightly floured surface and knead the dough until it is smooth and slightly elastic, about 5 minutes. Roll the dough into a ball and transfer it to a buttered bowl. Cover the bowl with plastic wrap and let it rest at room temperature for 20 minutes.
3. Divide the dough into 6 equal-size balls. Transfer 1 ball to a lightly floured surface (keep the other dough balls covered with a clean dish towel). Roll the dough into a 6-inch circle. Using a pastry brush, baste the surface of the dough with butter and sprinkle with nigella seeds, if using. Fold the dough in half, forming a semicircle. Brush the surface of the semicircle with butter; fold it in half again to form a triangle. Gently roll out the dough to a thickness slightly less than 1/4 inch.
4. Heat a large skillet over medium-low heat. Brush the surface of the paratha with butter and sprinkle with salt. Place the bread, butter-side down, into

[CONTINUED]

the skillet. Cook until the bread begins to bubble, 2 to 3 minutes. Brush the exposed surface of the bread with butter and sprinkle with salt. Flip the bread and cook until the underside is golden, 2 to 3 minutes. Transfer the bread to a plate. Repeat with the remaining dough, butter, and nigella seeds.

What Else?

- The beauty of these parathas is their butteriness. Without the copious amount, they would be leathery and heavy instead of rich and flaky. So please don't skimp on the butter here, or you will wonder why you bothered making these in the first place.

- These breads are marvelous with dips, especially the Stupendous Hummus on page 256.

- I've yet to figure out a way to successfully reheat leftover parathas, so eat them all up the day you make them and you won't be faced with this quandary. (The microwave makes them warm and pliable for about 30 seconds, after which they cool down and turn into cardboard, in case you were wondering.)

- The nigella seeds (also called black onion seeds) are purely optional, but they do give the dish a smoky, earthy flavor that I really like. Without them, the parathas are more kid-friendly and still delicious. Black or white sesame seeds or even poppy seeds would be a nice substitute. The flavor will be completely different, but still very tasty.

PISTACHIO SHORTBREAD

If I had a signature dish, it would be shortbread. Buttery, rich, crumbly short-bread is not only pretty much my favorite thing on earth to eat, it's also about the easiest thing a pastry cook can make. And I've made it in every possible variation I can think of, and as new ideas pop into my head, I will practically run to the kitchen to bake up those, too. Right now I've got a coconut curry shortbread idea floating around up there, and by the time I finish writing this chapter, I guarantee I'll have made it (if it's good, you can look for it in the next book).

This shortbread recipe is one of my all-time favorites, a classic and gorgeous combination of pistachio nuts and orange blossom water. It reminds me of Morocco, where I've never been but dream about in sweet, perfumed reveries. This shortbread is as close as I've come, but until the day I take the trip, it's not a bad recompense.

Makes 1 (8-inch) pan

2 cups all-purpose flour

3/4 cup confectioners' sugar

1/2 cup pistachios

3/4 teaspoon kosher salt

1 cup (2 sticks) chilled unsalted butter, cut into 1/2-inch cubes

2 teaspoons orange blossom water

1. Preheat the oven to 325°F.
2. Combine the flour, confectioners' sugar, pistachios, and salt in a food processor. Pulse until the nuts are coarsely to finely chopped. Pulse in the butter and orange blossom water until a moist ball forms.
3. Press the dough evenly into an 8-inch-square baking pan. Prick the short-bread all over with a fork. Bake the shortbread until barely golden, 45 to 50 minutes. Slice the shortbread while warm.

What Else?

The basic shortbread recipe sans the nuts and orange blossom water can be your blank canvas for all kinds of shortbread variations. Here are some:

• Leave it plain and simple, or even better, add the scraping of one fat, moist vanilla bean or a teaspoon of vanilla extract.

• Add any citrus zest along with a splash of the matching juice.

• Substitute any other nut for the pistachios.

• Use rose water or a nice, aged spirit for flavoring.

• Spices are marvelous. Add grated nutmeg, cinnamon, ginger, mace, cardamom, alone or in combination.

• Use up to half whole wheat flour. Sprinkling the top with Demerara sugar is a good addition here (or really, anywhere).

• Use the shortbread as a base for toffee cookies; as soon as it comes out of the oven, sprinkle with chopped bittersweet chocolate. Return to a turned-off but still hot oven for 5 minutes, then spread the chocolate flat with a spatula. Sprinkle with nuts and let the chocolate set before cutting.

FIGGY DEMERARA
SNACKING CAKE

One recent summer, *Saveur* magazine printed a recipe for a simple Hungarian sour cherry cake. Made with whole wheat flour, it was an easily mixed, flat, homey-looking cake with a deep, earthy taste that wasn't too sweet, riddled with little pockets of intensely jamlike sour cherries. The edges of the cake got a little singed in the oven while the center stayed soft. It was rustically beautiful and altogether delicious, and I made it several times during the short sour cherry window.

When the cherries were gone, I proceeded to make the cake with every fruit that came my way, but none was as good—until I found figs.

Or, more correctly, the figs found me, just as they do every September when the green and mauve fruit ripen on the tree in my backyard.

Usually I nibble my figs out of hand as quickly as I pick them. But this past year, the summer was so hot and so dry (apparently fig-happy conditions) that I got a bumper crop. There were more figs than even Dahlia and I could eat, and we really did try.

I gave some away to a few lucky friends, and decided to cook something with the rest—a luxury I hardly ever permitted myself in leaner years.

The first thing I made was this cake. I had tweaked the recipe already in prior experiments, so by the time the figs were ready to be cake, the cake was ready for them. Since the figs have less acid than the cherries, the cake was altogether sweeter and mellower, but just as appealing. I couldn't decide which version I like better. But since sour cherry season and fig season are months apart, there's plenty of room for both.

Serves 12 to 14

2 dozen fresh figs, halved lengthwise through the stem
2¼ cups whole wheat flour, plus more for the pan
1 cup (2 sticks) unsalted butter, softened, plus more for the pan

[CONTINUED]

1 1/4 cups granulated sugar

3 tablespoons brandy

1 teaspoon vanilla extract

1 large egg

1 tablespoon baking powder

1 teaspoon kosher salt

1 cup milk

2 tablespoons Demerara or raw sugar

1. Preheat the oven to 400°F. Toss the figs with 1/4 cup flour; set aside.
2. Grease an 18 × 13 × 1-inch baking sheet with butter and dust with flour; set aside. In a large bowl, beat together the butter, granulated sugar, brandy, and vanilla with a hand mixer on medium speed until pale and fluffy. Add the egg; beat until incorporated.
3. In a medium bowl, whisk together the remaining 2 cups whole wheat flour, baking powder, and salt. With the mixer running on low speed, alternately add the flour mixture and milk in 3 batches to make a batter. Spoon the batter onto the reserved baking sheet and smooth evenly. Nestle the figs into the batter evenly all over the top. Sprinkle with the Demerara sugar. Bake until the cake is golden brown, 45 to 50 minutes. Let the cake cool 30 minutes before serving.

What Else?

- I've made this with almost every kind of summer fruit I could get my hands on, and far and away the best ones, besides the figs, are sour cherries, nectarines, and plums. Peaches and blueberries are too mild tasting to stand up to the whole wheat flour, while raspberries are too juicy and blackberries too seedy. This said, every single one of those variation cakes got gobbled up entirely, so I might just be picky. If you want to substitute plums or sour cherries, use 2 pounds, weighed out before you pit them. The cherries can be used whole but you need to quarter or thickly slice the plums depending upon how large they are.

- This recipe makes a lot of cake, but it's not an easy recipe to scale down. I know, since I've tried it many times, and the halved cakes are never quite as good as the full recipe. I think it's because of the pan size. Something magical happens when the batter gets baked in that 1-inch-high pan. It gets a little crisp and browned around the edges, while the center bakes through and stays soft. In a small pan, it just doesn't work as well. In a 9×13-inch baking pan, with 2-inch-high sides, you don't get the same browning on the edges; instead the whole cake stays soft. And in a 9×13-inch sheet pan with 1-inch-high sides (also called a quarter sheet pan), the whole thing gets too brown too quickly. Plus there is the problem of halving 1 egg. While it can be done (whisk it in a bowl first, then just use half of it), it's one of those persnickety, pain-in-the-rear instructions that make me balk and that I wouldn't want to inflict on you. So make this for a party, or plan to give away loads to your neighbors, who will love you for it because it's an excellent cake.

Autumn

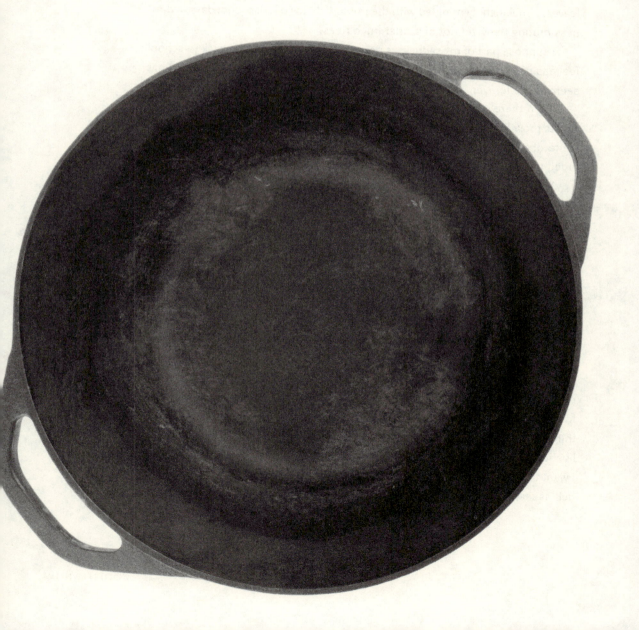

There is a mournful quality to the onset of autumn.

It's a mild ache that creeps up with the appearance of the first fallen leaves, a melancholy mingled with the immediate joy of crisp, cool days, a dimness muting the vivid riot of scarlet-hued trees.

I suppose part of my sadness is never having gotten over the back-to-school feelings of my childhood, when the freedom of summer melted away for what seemed like forever.

Then there is the change in the light. There is less of it, of course, as the nights grow longer. And the quality of light changes, too, going from the bright white of a blinding summer sun to a more subdued sepia hue, the color of faded photographs and pangs of nostalgia.

What pulls me out of this glum hole is the humming expectancy of the holiday season, which pretty much begins right after Labor Day and continues through the darkest months. This celebratory run often commences with an invitation to the very first we-are-staying-in-the-city-for-the-weekend cocktail party, then continues gleefully through Rosh Hashana, Halloween, Thanksgiving, Hanukkah, and Christmas, culminating on New Year's Eve, the mother of all holiday feasts, at which I always insist on serving caviar and Champagne to excess, even when it's just Daniel and me and a sleepy child, cuddled in the house watching obscure foreign films while the neighborhood bubbles and froths with excitement just outside the window.

Be it New Year's Eve or an intimate dinner gathering, parties bring light, music, friends, and food together into the chilly black nights. And for me, the food is at the heart of every get-together, no matter how casual. Even something as simple as inviting another couple with kids over for a midafternoon libation means I get to indulge in some menu planning, fantasizing about what I want to make, what to serve. Olives, clementines, the last of the season's fennel, sausages, and Sweet and Spicy Candied Nuts (page 365) will feed both children and their parents while the adults sip red wine, with freshly pressed apple cider for those small teetotalers in tow.

Fancier parties demand more elaborate fare and I'm happy to chop, toss, roast, and bake my way through windy afternoons. I've always thought of autumn as the season for elaborate cooking projects that happily eat up entire weekends—homemade puff pastry, for example, or canning jams and pickles. It's real, honest cooking, which no longer seems like sweaty work after the salads of summer. These are cozy endeavors that keep you close to the stove in the warmest room in the house.

This said, I have to admit that since I had my daughter, Dahlia, I'm less inclined toward multiday cooking projects, though I do like staying near the kitchen at all times.

The recipes I gravitate to are simple and hearty, homey and rustic: perhaps a pan of moist gingerbread studded with melting tart cranberries (page 339) or a farro pasta with spicy salami and tomatoes (page 325) to fuel Daniel's marathoning inclinations.

Dahlia's too young for school as of yet, but even so I love the lunchbox appeal of Whole Wheat Peanut Butter Sandies (page 314), and make them as much for my own afternoon snacking as for hers. And I love the way that braises (Braised Leg of Lamb with Garlicky Root Vegetable Puree, page 357), stews (Spicy Three-Meat Chili, page 330), and large pots of soup (Beet and Cabbage Borscht with Dill, page 348) simmer and perfume the house, warming the bones after cold rainy days.

Of course this urge to cook isn't just about keeping warm; it's also about taking advantage of the latest farmers' market offerings. Autumn, the traditional harvesting time of year, means abundance, especially of staunch keeping crops that used to fill root cellars back when people had them, feeding a family all winter long.

Without a place to store potatoes and turnips, I rely on the farmers to do that for me, and try not to buy those vegetables until as late in the season as possible. In October, I tend to cling to summer for as long as I can, still nibbling tomato sandwiches for lunch, ignoring sweet potatoes and pumpkins for weeks after their arrival. It's as if my refusal to embrace the cold-weather crops will forestall the inevitable deep freeze, will soften winter's eventual grasp.

But by the time the weather grows truly cold and I trade in my short leather jacket for a long and woolly overcoat, I've eased into the spirit enough to start embracing those hardy, dense-fleshed vegetables—waxy rutabagas, thick-skinned winter squash, verdant Brussels sprouts—all of which can benefit from plenty of soul-warming stove time to render them sweetly irresistible. Roasting is my go-to method for these, and it never fails me; as long as I add enough oil and salt to season them and turn them golden and caramelized, they always taste deep and rich and satisfying.

In fact, when I think of autumn foods, a scarred pan full of brown-edged roasted vegetables strewn with herbs is actually the image that leaps to mind. It's the colors—the ruddy shades of pumpkins, carrots, and yams that recall the leaves outside the window. Autumn is orange and gold and red, intense in flavor, opulent in color, festive in spirit. And even if it starts out rather shakily, at least as far as my mood is concerned, it always ends up bright, twinkling, and exceedingly well fed.

OCTOBER

CELERY SALAD WITH WALNUTS AND PARMESAN

When there's nothing else in the house to make into salad, I remember the celery.

It's always there when I need it to be, a neglected stalwart usually just waiting to be mixed up with tuna and mayo or sautéed into a soup. Sometimes I'll forget about it for weeks. But then, when I'm craving a salad and the greens in the fridge are sad and wilted in their bags, I'll slice up some crisp celery stalks, toss them with a little olive oil and lemon juice, and enjoy a quickly made, always available salad with a juicy fresh bite.

If I've got them on hand, sometimes I'll sprinkle a few walnuts into the salad bowl. The nuts add a different kind of crunch—a softer, buttery, rich crunch against the celery's watery, cold, snappy crunch. The two together are compelling, especially when topped with some shaved good Parmesan cheese to add a salty creaminess to the mix. I'll eat it all up, and think, *Why don't I make this more often?* It makes me happy every time.

Serves 4

1 cup walnuts
1 1/2 tablespoons red wine vinegar
1/2 teaspoon kosher salt
Freshly ground black pepper to taste
1/3 cup extra-virgin olive oil
8 large celery stalks with leaves, thinly sliced
2 ounces good Parmesan cheese, shaved

1. Preheat the oven to 350°F. Spread the walnuts in a single layer on a rimmed baking sheet. Toast, tossing once halfway through, until the nuts are golden, 7 to 10 minutes. Cool and coarsely chop.

2. In a small bowl, whisk together the vinegar, salt, and pepper; whisk in the

oil. Combine the walnuts, celery and leaves, and cheese in a large salad bowl. Add the vinaigrette and toss gently to combine.

What Else?

- This is the place to use that pricey chunk of imported-from-Italy Parmigiano-Reggiano cheese you picked up at the gourmet market. Its complex, salty flavor really adds a lot of depth to this otherwise very simple salad. But any aged cheese, such as Cheddar, Gouda, or manchego, can stand in nicely.

- If you are leaving the cheese out altogether, throw in a handful of drained capers or chop an anchovy into the vinaigrette to give the salad a saline kick. This is what I do when I make this to share with Daniel.

- Though I happen to judge celery as one of the vegetable kingdom's most underappreciated specimens, I know it's not for everyone. In that case, you could try this with julienned or thinly shaved fennel, which has a similar texture and a deep, sweet, anise flavor.

- I can easily polish off a big bowl of salad without any help, but if you're wondering what you might serve this with, I can picture it as a nice accompaniment to a ploughman's supper, with some pickles, crusty bread, sliced sausages or ham, and/or hard-cooked eggs.

CUMIN SEED ROASTED CAULIFLOWER WITH SALTED YOGURT, MINT, AND POMEGRANATE SEEDS

When the nights turn blustery and the temperature drops, I know that roasted vegetable season has arrived, and I embrace it with reckless abandon. I'll roast any kind of sturdy vegetable that I can cut up and fit into my oven, but one of my favorites is cauliflower, preferably tossed with whole cumin seeds. Not only does the cumin act as a natural remedy to help reduce the dreaded intestinal gas factor (or so I've been told), but it also adds a pleasant earthy flavor to balance the assertive tang of the vegetable.

Roasted cauliflower with cumin makes a nice and simple side dish. Even Dahlia will eat it if she's distracted enough. But recently I made it into lunch. I roasted up a small head all for myself, and added a topping of salted yogurt (which is simply a good, full-fat yogurt with a little kosher salt mixed in), a few leftover pomegranate seeds (which I can buy at my local market already picked out of the husk), and a smattering of bright green chopped fresh mint. It was a perfect light lunch. It could even be dinner, served over brown rice, bulgur, or some other filling, toasty grain, for a warming meal to start out roasting season right.

1 large head cauliflower, cut into bite-size florets

Serves 2

2 tablespoons extra-virgin olive oil

1 teaspoon whole cumin seeds

1/2 teaspoon kosher salt, plus additional

1/2 teaspoon freshly ground black pepper

Plain yogurt, for serving

Chopped fresh mint leaves, for serving

Pomegranate seeds, for serving

1. Preheat the oven to 425°F. Toss the cauliflower with the oil, cumin seeds, salt, and pepper. Spread the mixture in an even layer on a large baking sheet. Roast, tossing occasionally, until the cauliflower is tender and its edges are toasty, 20 to 30 minutes.
2. Whisk a pinch of salt into the yogurt. Dollop the yogurt on top of the cauliflower and strew the mint and pomegranate seeds over the yogurt.

What Else?

- Don't worry if your florets seem unevenly cut. The bigger pieces will get tender and golden, while the little bits get crispy-caramelized all over. I think it makes for an excellent contrast of textures.

- I abhor the chalky texture of low-fat yogurts, so please use full-fat for this dish. The only exception I've found is 2 percent plain Greek yogurt, which tastes more or less like the real deal.

- If you don't have pomegranate seeds, just leave them off. The dish is lovely enough without them.

RAW KALE SALAD WITH ANCHOVY-DATE DRESSING

A few years ago I made a raw kale salad, a recipe I adapted from Franny's restaurant in Brooklyn and subsequently published in my column in the *New York Times*.

Filled with tangy pecorino, loads of pungent garlic, and salty crisp bread crumbs, it became one of my favorite things in the world to eat—and I ate it as often as I could.

The great thing about the kale salad is that it's ideal for entertaining. I could make it a few hours in advance and it would hold up during the whole party, wilting a little but getting even tastier as it sat. It could last for hours—if it didn't get devoured first, that is.

The only thing I didn't like about the salad was that my husband Daniel, who doesn't eat cheese, couldn't partake. This limited the occasions I could serve it.

Then one day, while I was making a Daniel-friendly date-citrus-anchovy dressing to toss with arugula for a friend's party, I got the idea to use kale instead.

The slightly sticky, pungent date dressing was delicious, but it always wilted the arugula minutes after being dressed. Kale, however, would stand up to the dressing, and the whole thing seemed like it would be a nice, cheeseless alternative to my usual mix.

It worked beautifully, with the sweetness of the dates and salty, funky tang of the anchovies mitigating the assertive, green flavor of the kale. The salad was wonderful from the moment it graced the table, and then proceeded to get better as the evening wore on, softening, deepening, and becoming even more interesting and complex with the passing hours—the perfect guest at any party.

6 to 8 large medjool dates, pitted, smashed, and finely chopped

6 anchovy fillets, finely chopped

3 garlic cloves, finely chopped

Finely grated zest of 2 oranges

Finely grated zest of 2 lemons

½ cup extra-virgin olive oil

1 tablespoon plus 1 teaspoon red wine vinegar, more to taste

2 large or 3 small bunches Tuscan kale, ribs removed

Coarse sea salt, if needed

1. In a medium bowl, stir together the dates (use more dates if you like a sweeter salad and fewer if you prefer a less sweet salad), anchovies, garlic, orange zest, and lemon zest. Stir in the olive oil and vinegar.
2. Wash and dry the kale leaves; stack the leaves and slice them thinly cross-wise. Transfer the greens to a large salad bowl. Add the vinaigrette and toss gently to combine. Add salt and more vinegar if needed

What Else?

*   Russian red kale works well here, too, if you can't find Tuscan (aka laci-nato, black, or dinosaur kale). Regular green curly kale is a last choice because the leaves tend to be tough, but it will work if you slice it thinly enough.

*   Kale leaves toughen as they age, so it's best if you make this dish with the most tender bunches you can find. That's not to say that you can't use kale that's on the older side (because, well, I have). Just slice it very finely before tossing it with the vinaigrette.

*   Although I haven't done this yet, I would bet a princely sum that this dress-ing would be amazing on roasted or steamed cauliflower.

[CONTINUED]

- When Meyer lemons are in season, you can substitute their zest in full for the orange and lemon zest.

- By the way, try to use the zested citrus in the next few days, as it tends to harden up pretty quickly when denuded of the protective, oily skin. You can juice the lemons and freeze the juice. I usually end up eating the oranges almost immediately, but you can juice and freeze them, too. Or use them to make a citrus salad, such as a variation on the Cara Cara orange salad on page 54.

ROASTED BLACKFISH WITH OLIVES AND SAGE

If you're not the type of cook who reels in her own catch, fish names make very little sense. You look at all the steaks and fillets spread out on the ice, and contemplate their names: red snapper, bluefish, rainbow trout, yellow fin, black bass. They sound wonderfully exotic and colorful. But in fact, except for tuna, salmon, and artic char, they are all some shade of white or tan, with nothing red, blue, yellow, or rainbow-hued about them.

And so it is with blackfish, a plump, pinkish-white fillet that I caught sight of at the fish stand at the farmers' market one day a few years back.

I'd never heard of blackfish before, but I liked the look of the thick, pearly fillets, each one large enough to feed two. A quick check on my Monterey Bay Aquarium phone app confirmed that they were sustainable, so I brought a large piece with me for dinner that night.

I cooked it simply, sautéing it in a little butter and lemon, and savored the fish's sweet ocean flavor, which was mild but very succulent. Since then, I've cooked blackfish every which way I can think of—seared, grilled, broiled, and roasted—and it is always good. As long as I don't overcook it (in which case it turns mushy and falls apart), blackfish will adapt itself to my fishy whims.

And for a while, my whim was roasting. I love roasting fish because it's easy, only dirties one pan, and tends not to stink up the house as much as, say, stove-top grilling.

You can season roasted fish with almost anything or with practically nothing. As long as the fish is fresh, it will always taste good.

In this recipe, take the middle road, topping a couple of fillets with a little lemon, some earthy sage, and some sliced black olives that shrivel in the oven and give the mellow fish a perky, chewy, salty bite. In fact, the olives are the only black thing about this dish, which is also a little browned around the edges, dark green from the sage, and moon-white, of course, from the blackfish.

3 tablespoons extra-virgin olive oil

2 (1-pound) skin-on blackfish fillets, patted dry

Kosher salt, for seasoning

Freshly ground black pepper, for seasoning

1 small bunch fresh sage

1/2 cup chopped pitted kalamata or other olives

Freshly squeezed juice of 1/2 lemon

Urfa or Aleppo red pepper, for seasoning

Best-quality extra-virgin olive oil, for drizzling (optional)

1. Preheat the oven to 425°F. Drizzle 1 tablespoon oil into the bottom of a baking sheet. Arrange the fish fillets, skin-side down, in the pan. Season the fish generously with salt and pepper. Tear the sage leaves into small pieces and sprinkle over the fish. Scatter the olives on top of and around the fish. Drizzle the fish with the remaining 2 tablespoons oil.

2. Transfer the pan to the oven and roast until the fish is just opaque, 8 to 10 minutes. Squeeze lemon juice over the fish and dust the fillet with Turkish (Urfa) or Aleppo pepper. Finish with a light drizzle of good oil, if desired.

What Else?

- If blackfish (also called tautog) isn't readily available near you, you can use the same technique with other fish (striped bass, sea bass, mackerel), though you might have to adjust the roasting time, depending upon the thickness of the fillets.

- One of these days I am going to try this with some finely chopped preserved lemon instead of the olives. If you beat me to it, a few tablespoons will probably do.

- If you don't have or would rather not use sage (it does have a musky pronounced flavor that not everyone loves), substitute rosemary or thyme branches.

- Green olives give this dish a completely different flavor than the rich, soft black ones. They are brighter and zestier, and just lovely.

- I love to serve roasted fish with roasted potatoes, because I can cook everything in the oven at more or less the same time. The roasted sweet potatoes with cinnamon (page 302) make a terrific side dish here, and you can start them in the oven before adding the fish for the last 8 minutes or so, then take everything out together and serve at once.

A Dish by Another Name

- To make Blackfish with Roasted Sweet Peppers and Olives, thinly slice 2 red, yellow, or orange bell peppers (or two different colors). Toss with oil and salt and spread out on a baking sheet. Roast, stirring once or twice, in a 375°F oven for 20 to 30 minutes, until soft and light brown around the edges. Place the seasoned, oiled fish on top, sprinkle with olives, and continue to roast until the fish is just cooked through, about 10 minutes. Serve the peppers over the fish, with chopped herbs if you like.

CINNAMON ROASTED SWEET POTATOES AND GARLIC

As soon as the first new crop of sweet potatoes hits the market stands, I bring a couple home to roast up until the tubers turn honeyed and velvety and just beg for a knob of butter or a drizzle of good olive oil to set off their plush orange flesh.

These days there are dozens of sweet potato varieties floating around the market, and I've tried as many as I see, including gentle white sweet potatoes, richly sweet red jewel yams, and tiny baby sweet potatoes with delicate skins. All of them have their charms, but my favorites are the so-called garnet yams, which arrive in the market in October, then disappear right after Christmas like a fleeting, edible gift.

I usually bake my sweet potatoes plain with just oil and salt. They really don't need any other embellishment. But last year, after successfully roasting some Yukon Gold potatoes with a broken-up cinnamon stick and unpeeled garlic cloves strewn on the top, I decided to apply that same method to my pretty garnet sweets. It was one of those suddenly obvious, why-haven't-I-done-this-before combinations. The cinnamon added that familiar, autumnal scent that made the sweet potatoes taste like Thanksgiving, while the garlic lent a caramelized, candy-like note that was about a million times tastier than marshmallows—at least if you ask me.

1½ pounds sweet potatoes, preferably garnet yams, peeled and
    cut into 1-inch chunks
6 unpeeled garlic cloves
3 tablespoons olive oil
2 thyme branches
1 cinnamon stick, broken into pieces
1 teaspoon kosher salt
½ teaspoon freshly ground black pepper

Serves 4

1. Preheat the oven to 425°F. Put all the ingredients in a baking pan and toss to combine, then spread out in an even layer.
2. Roast until the potatoes are tender and browned, 25 to 45 minutes. Serve hot or warm, along with the garlic cloves.

What Else?

• I love how the cinnamon stick subtly imbues the potatoes with a touch of sweetness, but you could take it in other directions flavorwise. A bay leaf and a sprinkling of smoked paprika would be nice and savory, or you could just roast the potatoes and garlic and season them with sage salt (page 337) when they come out of the oven.

• Make sure everyone squeezes the rich, caramelized garlic paste out of the skins to eat with the potatoes. It makes the dish.

• If your family can't embrace the notion of sweet potatoes without a sticky glaze on top, drizzle a little honey over the potatoes about halfway through baking.

• For a spicy, zippy flavor, add a large pinch of crushed red pepper flakes to the mix.

STIR-FRIED CHICKEN WITH LEEKS, OYSTER MUSHROOMS, AND PEANUTS

As much as I've loved take-out Chinese food—the cheap, filling, completely inauthentic stuff I used to have delivered from my neighborhood joint on a regular basis—I recently gave it up. I've become horrified by what I assume is a meal comprised of factory farm chicken and CAFO beef. Not to say I'm a total purist when it comes to meats, but giving up meaty stir-fries in take-out Chinese? That I can do.

So these days, when I get a hankering for inauthentic Chinese food, I scratch the itch by making it myself.

And here's what I've learned, something I've long known in theory but never really lived: Stir-fries are easy. They are quick. The hardest part is cutting up the ingredients but once that is done, dinner practically is, too.

In this recipe, I use humanely raised boneless chicken thighs (breasts also work if you like white meat) marinated in soy sauce, rice wine vinegar, and sesame oil to give it a deep, nutty flavor. Then I add mushrooms and leeks to the pan as the vegetable factor. (Stir-fries always need a vegetable factor.) Mushrooms work especially well because they add a meaty character that deepens the flavor of the chicken. Then I garnish everything with loads of chopped peanuts for crunch and a shower of cilantro for a fresh, herby flavor. Together they help make a dish that's a cut above the usual takeout, in so many ways.

Serves 2 to 3

2 tablespoons soy sauce (less if you are using dark soy or tamari, which are stronger)

2 tablespoons rice wine vinegar, plus additional for serving

1½ tablespoons toasted (Asian) sesame oil

2 teaspoons light brown sugar (or granulated sugar)

¾ pound boneless, skinless chicken meat (you can use either breast or thigh), cut crosswise into ½-inch strips

2 tablespoons finely chopped fresh gingerroot

2 garlic cloves, finely chopped

3 tablespoons peanut oil

½ pound oyster mushrooms, sliced ½ inch thick

2 to 3 leeks, white and light green parts only, cleaned and thinly sliced

Pinch kosher salt (optional)

3 tablespoons finely chopped peanuts, for serving

2 tablespoons chopped fresh cilantro, for serving

Steamed rice, for serving

1. In a small bowl, whisk together the soy sauce, vinegar, sesame oil, and brown sugar. In a large bowl, combine the chicken with half the marinade (reserve the other half for stir-frying) and half the chopped ginger and garlic. Cover the chicken with plastic wrap and refrigerate for at least 30 minutes and up to 2 hours (longer than that and the chicken will get mushy).

2. Heat a large 12-inch or so skillet over the highest heat until the pan is screaming hot, about 5 minutes. Add 1 tablespoon peanut oil and tilt the skillet so that the bottom is evenly covered with oil. Lift the chicken from the marinade (shake off any excess liquid) and add to the hot skillet. Cook, stirring constantly and quickly, until the chicken is just cooked through, about 2 minutes for breasts and 3 to 4 minutes for thigh meat. Transfer the chicken to a plate.

3. Add the remaining peanut oil to the skillet. Add the mushrooms and cook, stirring constantly, until the mushrooms are browned and soft, 2 to 3 minutes. Add the leeks and cook until wilted, about 1 minute. Stir in the reserved marinade. Push the vegetables to the border of the pan, leaving an open space in the middle. Add the remaining chopped ginger and garlic to the open space. Mash it around with your spoon until it is tender and fragrant, about 30 seconds. Return the chicken to the pan and quickly toss it with the ginger, garlic, and vegetables. Taste and add a pinch of salt if it needs it.

4. Remove the pan from the heat and toss in the peanuts and cilantro. Mound the stir-fry over steamed rice, and sprinkle judiciously with rice wine vinegar before serving.

What Else?

- You might wonder why I use a skillet rather than a wok for a stir-fry recipe. I actually sold my wok at my annual stoop sale years ago. Traditional Chinese woks in China (or Chinese restaurants) have a special, double-ringed burner that allows for adjusting the flame high enough to lap the sides of the pan. Western stoves don't have that feature and just can't get a wok that hot. Trust me—your heaviest straight-sided skillet will retain more heat and produce better stir-fries at home.

- Here I used about the same amount of meat to vegetables, but one of the reasons I like stir-fries is that they are an easy way to play with the meat-to-vegetable proportions on your plate without other people really noticing. If I'm in the mood for plenty of veggies (which is most of the time), I'll let them dominate the stir-fry.

- This dish serves two, mainly because I was just cooking for Daniel and myself (plus a wee portion for Dahlia). But if you are trying to cook for four to six, just double the recipe and cook everything in two batches (if you overcrowd the skillet, the meat won't sear properly). It comes together so quickly that both batches will make it to the table piping hot.

- Another good reason to double this recipe is to have leftovers. The flavors only improve overnight, although I would make a fresh batch of rice or serve it over quinoa or millet. Rice is just never the same after day one, even when heated up in the microwave.

- If you're not a mushroom fan or just want something emerald green in your stir-fry, you can substitute nearly any green vegetable. Sturdy ones such as broccoli and snow peas benefit from being blanched for a minute or two before hitting the wok, but tender leafy greens—bok choy, spinach, kale, a late season stray zucchini or green pepper—can all be added raw.

CARROTY MAC AND CHEESE

Like most little kids, Dahlia loves macaroni and cheese, and I've made it for her in many guises, running the gamut of techniques. My aim is always the same—to make the dish quickly with a minimum of fuss, and to use a maximum of vegetables that she will tolerate and not pick out.

This is one of both our favorites. It's comforting, crusty topped, soft centered, and very cheesy—but not at all sophisticated. Just simple, kid-friendly homemade food with the added grown-up appeal of lots of healthful carrots tossed into the mix.

I got the idea from a chef's recipe in a glossy food magazine. The chef called for cooking carrots in butter and orange juice, pureeing them, and using the puree as a sauce for mac and cheese. I tried the recipe as written and was disappointed. It was a lot of work and I didn't like the sweetness of the citrus fruit interfering with my cheesy goodness.

So I decided to come up with my own simplified and ultra-Cheddary version. It was a huge hit with the under-three crowd and their parents, too.

It's a straightforward recipe that comes together without much fuss, other than having to grate some carrots. But to make up for that, I've eliminated the need to make a cheese sauce on the top of the stove. Instead, I toss the hot pasta with grated Cheddar, butter, sour cream for creaminess, and eggs to hold it all together. The grated carrots get boiled along with the pasta, so cooking them isn't an extra step. And the tiny orange shreds look so much like the Cheddar that your kids might not even notice they are there. Dahlia certainly hasn't, and while I've never lied to her about their inclusion, I might have left out the word *carrot* in the dish description—accidentally, of course.

Serves 6

2 cups whole wheat macaroni

2½ cups coarsely grated carrots (about 8 small)

3 cups grated sharp Cheddar cheese

¼ cup (½ stick) unsalted butter, cut into pieces

[CONTINUED]

¾ cup sour cream

¼ cup whole milk

2 large eggs

1 teaspoon kosher salt

¾ teaspoon mustard powder

¼ teaspoon freshly ground black pepper

¼ cup finely grated Parmesan cheese

1. Preheat the oven to 400°F and grease an 8-inch-square baking pan. Arrange a rack in the top third of the oven.

2. Cook the macaroni according to the package instructions in a large pot of boiling salted water. Add the carrots 3 minutes before the pasta is finished cooking; drain well.

3. While the pasta is hot, stir in all but ½ cup of the Cheddar and the butter. In a bowl, whisk together the sour cream, milk, eggs, salt, mustard powder, and pepper. Fold the mixture into the pasta.

4. Scrape the mixture into the prepared pan. Sprinkle the remaining Cheddar and the Parmesan over the top. Bake until the casserole is firm to the touch and golden brown, about 30 minutes.

What Else?

- If you're grating your Cheddar cheese in the food processor, you don't have to wash out the machine before grating the carrots. Or vice versa.

- This is one of those macaroni and cheeses with an eggy custard base that puffs as it cooks, and is cut into squares to serve, like a casserole, as opposed to that gooey, creamy, stove-top béchamel sauce version. I know that some people have strong opinions about proper mac and cheese (I'm an equal opportunist myself), but I thought I'd let you know what you're getting.

- Feed this dish to the kids as is; grown-ups should indulge with a squirt of fiery Sriracha or other hot sauce all over the top.

- You can vary the cheese to give this rather plain (if tasty) dish more personality. Gruyère, aged Cheddar, pecorino, and aged Gouda will all add a sophisticated allure that will raise it above mere kids' food.

A Dish by Another Name

- To make Quick and Homey Mac and Cheese: Cook 1 cup of macaroni in a small pot of salted water according to the package instructions (the whole wheat takes about 10 minutes). Drain the macaroni, then add it back to the pot, and over low heat, stir in 1/2 cup grated Cheddar, 2 tablespoons heavy cream, and a pinch of salt. Cook, stirring, over low heat for 2 to 3 minutes until the cheese and cream are blended in and creamy.

SPINACH SALAD WITH DRIED CRANBERRIES AND PINE NUTS

At first glance, this salad might seem like one of those classic things you've seen maybe a few too many times before. You know, the kind of dish you'd read about on a menu, yawn, and order something else.

But one bite will convince you that this recipe really is something different, and better than those other namby-pamby salads you've seen before. That's because this one is a tightly orchestrated cascade of flavors balancing the pungency of the garlic and anchovy paste with the fruity tartness of dried cranberries and the sweet complexity of the sherry vinegar. It's the kind of salad that salad haters tend to devour because there is so much more going on than just oil, vinegar, and leaves.

It's the perfect thing to serve as a dinner party first course, when people expect a fancy salad with an array of colors and textures but one that isn't too filling to ruin the meal ahead.

Although you can make this salad with the bags of baby spinach you see at the supermarket (and I've done it that way plenty of times), if you can get a bunch of good, crinkly, mature spinach, preferably from the farmers' market, use that instead. Mature spinach is hardier and thicker than the baby leaves, and won't wilt as easily. Plus older, wiser spinach has a much deeper, earthier, and I think more interesting and profound flavor than those meek little tykes. And since these days no one seems to be using a lot of mature spinach in salads, it will lessen the been-there, done-that factor to nearly nil.

1/4 cup pine nuts
1 garlic clove, finely chopped
1 anchovy fillet, chopped
Kosher salt and freshly ground black pepper to taste
2 1/2 teaspoons sherry vinegar
3 tablespoons extra-virgin olive oil

Serves 2 to 4

6 ounces spinach leaves, trimmed (about 8 cups)

¼ cup dried cranberries

1. In a small skillet, toast the pine nuts over medium heat until they turn golden and smell toasty, about 3 minutes. Pour them onto a plate to cool.
2. Place the garlic, anchovy, a pinch of salt, and black pepper in a mortar and pestle. Crush to form a paste (alternatively you can mash them together using the side of a knife). Transfer the paste to a small bowl. Whisk in the vinegar, then slowly whisk in the oil.
3. Place the spinach in a large bowl; add the vinaigrette and toss well to combine. Add the nuts and cranberries. Toss once more and serve.

What Else?

• Other nuts can stand in for the pine nuts, which can be hard to find and on the pricey side. I love slivered almonds, which have a similar mild flavor and soft crunch, but hazelnuts, pecans, and walnuts are also wonderful.

• Sometimes I add a pinch of red pepper flakes to zip this salad up.

• Dried cherries, chopped dried apricots or pears, or raisins can replace the dried cranberries. The object is to give the tangy dish a dash of sweetness, and there are many ways to get there.

• Arugula is a fine substitute for the spinach.

BROWN BUTTER MAPLE ROASTED PEARS

This is yet another variation on a honey-roasted pear recipe I stole—I mean, adapted—from the genius pastry chef Claudia Fleming of The North Fork Table and Inn. Years ago, when Claudia was the pastry chef at Gramercy Tavern and I was a newly minted freelancer for the *New York Times*, I helped her write her cookbook *The Last Course*. I think it's a wonderful book, and not just because I had a hand in writing it. It's because Claudia is brilliant at both technique and combining flavors, and that shines through in every recipe.

In Claudia's original roasted pear dish, she cooks the pears in rich, dark chestnut honey, then finishes them with butter and fresh thyme. In my version I swap out smoky Grade B maple syrup for the musky honey and brown the butter, which adds an autumnal, nutty complexity.

You can serve these with whipped cream on top of pound cake, or with little crisp cookies on the side. (The Pistachio Shortbread on page 281 would be ideal.) All of those things would be delightful. But all the pears really need for maximum enjoyment is a spoon. A bowl wouldn't hurt either.

3 almost-ripe Bosc or Anjou pears (1½ pounds), or a mixture of the two

¼ cup (½ stick) unsalted butter

⅔ cup maple syrup

1 cinnamon stick

⅛ teaspoon kosher salt

¾ teaspoon freshly squeezed lemon juice

Serves 6

1. Preheat the oven to 375°F. Peel the pears and halve them lengthwise. Use a melon baller or spoon to scoop out the core.
2. In a large skillet, melt 3 tablespoons butter over medium-high heat. Cook until frothy. Reduce the heat to medium and cook until the milk solids sink to the bottom of the pan and turn a nutty brown, 5 to 7 minutes. Brown

butter can burn quickly, so watch it carefully. Add the pears, cut-side down, to the pan. Cook, without moving, until the undersides are golden, about 3 minutes. Flip the pears and cook, without moving, 3 minutes more.

3. Pour the syrup over the pan and drop in the cinnamon stick. Flip the pears again and transfer the skillet to the oven. Bake until the pears are just tender, 10 to 12 minutes.

4. Use a slotted spoon to transfer the pears to a plate. Return the skillet to the heat. Add the salt. Simmer over medium-high heat until the sauce is syrupy, 3 to 5 minutes. Whisk in the remaining tablespoon butter and the lemon juice. Spoon the sauce over the pears and serve.

What Else?

• I wasn't trying to be nitpicky when I called for almost-ripe pears. If they are rock-hard, they won't have enough of that musky pear flavor; and if they are ripe, they will fall apart while cooking. So look for pears that just barely yield to pressure when you squeeze them.

• I always use Grade B maple syrup in cooking and baking. It is darker and more richly flavored than Grade A syrup. It's also widely available these days, but if you don't have any or can't find it for some reason, Grade A works nearly as well.

• Honey is an excellent stand-in for the maple syrup if you prefer it.

• Toasted nuts accentuate the nuttiness in the butter and add crunch. Pecans are my favorite to sprinkle on top here.

• Vanilla ice cream, crème fraîche, sour cream, fluffy fresh ricotta—this dish loves dairy products, and so do I.

WHOLE WHEAT PEANUT BUTTER SANDIES

Of all the birthday presents Dahlia got when she turned two—the books and stuffed animals, the plastic Three Little Pigs game complete with mean old wolf, the adorable BPA-free tea set—the gift that I enjoyed the most was a little paper bag filled with crumbly, brittle, lightly salted peanut butter cookies from her friend Alice's mama, Anna.

To be honest, after all the cupcakes, ice cream, and tortilla chips Dahlia ate at her party, I have to admit that I didn't actually share those cookies with her at all, but tucked them away in the back of a kitchen drawer to be savored by us grown-ups after bedtime disposed of the child.

Not that there was anything unwholesome about them. Anna, who is, incidentally, the pastry chef at Al Di La in Brooklyn (one of my favorite Italian restaurants in the city), made them with whole wheat flour, natural peanut butter, raw sugar, and eggs, and they were about as good for you as a cookie can be—a cookie made with sugar, that is. I just wanted to give Dahlia a few days to recover from her party before feeding her any more sugar. And by that time they were gone.

Naturally I felt very guilty about eating her present, so I set about righting the wrong by making another batch. Anna nicely gave me the recipe and I made them as soon as I could. My cookies were slightly more porous and lighter than Anna's, probably because of the different brands of peanut butter we used. But they were just as tasty. And Dahlia adored them—not that she had anything to compare them to. But just because they are good.

11/4 cups whole wheat pastry flour

1 teaspoon baking soda

1/4 teaspoon plus a pinch kosher salt

1/2 cup (1 stick) unsalted butter, softened

1/2 cup natural salted peanut butter

Makes about
42 cookies

1 cup Demerara or raw sugar

1 large egg

1 teaspoon pure vanilla extract

1. In a large bowl, sift together the flour, baking soda, and salt.
2. In the bowl of an electric mixer fitted with the paddle attachment, cream the butter. Beat in the peanut butter until smooth. Add the sugar and beat well. Beat in the egg and vanilla until fully incorporated. Stop and scrape down the bowl. Slowly beat in the dry ingredients.
3. Transfer the dough to a large sheet of plastic wrap or wax paper. Shape the dough into a 12-inch-long log. Wrap the dough in the plastic, using the wrap to help form the most uniform-size log possible. Transfer the dough to the refrigerator and chill at least 2 hours.
4. When you are ready to bake the cookies, preheat the oven to 350°F. Slice the dough into 1/4-inch-thick rounds and transfer them to an ungreased baking sheet 1 inch apart. Bake the cookies until lightly colored and semi-firm, about 15 minutes; rotate the sheets halfway through baking. Transfer the cookies to a wire rack to cool completely.

What Else?

- If you can't get salted peanut butter (and I feel very sorry for you if you can't, because unsalted peanut butter tastes like paste), use a heaping 1/2 teaspoon salt, or even 3/4 teaspoon salt, in these cookies. They need the salt.

- If you can't get coarse raw sugar, use regular brown sugar here. The texture of the cookie will be slightly denser and chewier but still highly delectable.

- For added texture and sugar content, roll the logs in more Demerara sugar before slicing and baking.

- I've never done it, but I'll bet almond butter would make a great substitute for the peanut butter here. If you try it, let me know how it goes.

NOVEMBER

HAM BONE, GREENS, AND BEAN SOUP

I've made ham hock soup, I've made bacon soup, and I've made soup with a diced-up pig's ear. But I doubt I would ever have made ham bone soup if I hadn't taken a liking to the name, which I spotted while flipping through an old Junior League cookbook one day.

The soup sounded so . . . well, bare bones, which intrigued me, as I imagined a pot swirling with nothing but water and several cartoonish white bones in it, the bony version of stone soup.

And just as stone soup is actually made of vegetables, so is ham bone soup. Most recipes call for beans, greens, onions, carrots—ingredients that would make any soup taste good, with or without the bones and stones.

However, unlike the stone in stone soup, which adds nothing to the vegetables in the pot, the ham bone makes the soup. It not only benefits from the bone's meaty, smoky flavor, but the broth gains body and richness from all the luscious marrow.

It's an excellent soup, flavorful, rich, easy to make, and filled with tender beans and an array of seasonal vegetables that you can vary with what's available. But no matter what you do, strive to include the cabbage, which, cooked for almost an hour, softens into translucent, marrow-imbued bits that melt on the tongue.

Serves 6 to 8

1 cup dried pinto beans

4 strips bacon, cut into 1/2-inch pieces

3 large carrots, peeled and diced

2 celery stalks, trimmed and diced

1 large onion, peeled and diced

3 garlic cloves, finely chopped

1 ham bone (11/4 pounds), cut into half or thirds (ask your butcher
   to do this for you)

1 bay leaf

2½ teaspoons salt, plus additional to taste

½ head green cabbage, shredded (about 8 cups)

1 bunch kale, stems removed and leaves chopped into bite-size pieces

Freshly ground black pepper to taste

Hot sauce or cider vinegar, for serving

1. Soak the beans in plenty of cold water overnight. If you don't have that much time, you can use the quick-soak method: In a large pot, bring the beans and plenty of cold water to a boil. Turn off the heat, cover the pot, and let stand for 1 hour. Drain the beans.

2. Heat a large pot over medium-high heat. Add the bacon and cook until crisp, 5 to 7 minutes; remove with a slotted spoon to a paper towel–lined plate and save for garnishing the soup. Add the carrots, celery, and onion to the bacon fat in the pan. Cook, stirring, until softened, about 5 minutes. Add the garlic and cook 1 minute.

3. Drop the ham bone and bay leaf into the pot and add 8 cups water and 2 ½ teaspoons salt. Bring the mixture to a boil over high heat; add the beans, reduce the heat to medium-low, and simmer for 30 minutes. Stir in the cabbage and simmer 30 minutes. Stir in the kale and simmer until the kale is soft but still vibrantly green, about 15 minutes. If you're like me, you'll want to remove the meat and delicious fatty bits from the ham bone, chop them up, and stir them back into the soup. Season with pepper, a dash of hot sauce or vinegar, and more salt, if needed. Crumble the reserved bacon on top.

What Else?

- If you don't see ham bones in your butcher's case, just ask; they will most likely have them stashed in the back. Ask your butcher to cut the bone in half or thirds for you, so it will easily fit into your pot. Plus cutting through the bone exposes all the good, rich marrow, allowing it to seep into the broth to give it a silky body and incomparable richness.

[CONTINUED]

- Ham bone is my number one choice for this soup, but I've made it with ham hocks, smoked pork shanks, and other various smoked pork bits on offer at the farmers' market. You could probably make it with smoked turkey necks or wings, too, though obviously the flavor will be different.

- If you want to make this soup without having to track down smoked pork parts, you can. Use the bacon as called for, then substitute chicken broth for the water. It will have great flavor if less body.

- If you want to substitute canned beans, give them a good rinse, then add them along with the cabbage. You will need about 2 cans (3 cups).

- Speaking of beans, I made this with all different kinds of beans before I decided that I loved the creaminess of pintos best against the brawny pork flavor. But it doesn't really matter what kind of beans you use so long as you like them.

- I can never get enough of kale, but collards, Swiss chard, or spinach (add it during the last 5 minutes of cooking) would be tasty in its place.

BUTTERNUT SQUASH RISOTTO
WITH PISTACHIOS AND LEMON

At our house, carbo-loading for the 2010 New York City marathon began with this autumnal risotto a few days before the big race. Daniel wanted something that combined plenty of carbs and vegetables, and I was in the mood to play with one of the season's carotenoid-heavy, orange-hued offerings, perhaps pumpkin, winter squash, or sweet potato. So I gave Daniel a choice between sweet potato gnocchi, pumpkin ravioli, or butternut squash risotto. Had he opted for gnocchi or ravioli, that's the recipe you'd be reading right now. But he chose risotto and I was excited to make it.

I'd never made butternut squash risotto before that night and wasn't exactly sure how to go about it. My first thought was to roast the squash and then stir the resulting puree into the risotto along with the broth. But that seemed like an awful lot of work for what was going to be a weeknight dinner.

A little bit of Web surfing yielded recipes that called for dicing the squash and sautéing it with the rice.

I liked the idea of sautéing the squash with the rice, but I didn't love the thought of dicing it. Shredding it in the food processor sounded easier. Plus the shreds, I hoped, would break apart and melt into the rice, forming a velvety sauce.

As I stood over the stove stirring the rice and squash, I thought about the garnishes. I had already pictured a dusting of chopped green pistachio nuts because I knew the color would be pretty, and I hoped the gentle crunch would be pleasant against the soft rice. But I also wanted something tart and bracing to lift the starchy rice out of its carbohydrate depths. My first impulse was to sprinkle on some balsamic vinegar (which I'm sure would also be good), but in the end, I decided to go with lemon and lemon zest for the purest, lightest flavor without the distracting caramel notes of the vinegar.

Daniel ate a double portion for dinner and leftovers for lunch the next

[CONTINUED]

afternoon before following up the risotto with spicy salami pasta (page 325) the night before the big day. And he flew through the race in under three hours. I'm perfectly aware of the months of physical and mental training it took for him to meet this goal. But if anyone asked, I gave his prerace carboloading full credit for his speedy success.

Serves 4 to 6

1/2 pound peeled butternut squash
About 6 cups chicken or vegetable stock
3 tablespoons unsalted butter
1 medium leek, thinly sliced
1 garlic clove, finely chopped
2 cups arborio rice
2 rosemary branches
3/4 teaspoon kosher salt, more to taste
1/3 cup dry white wine
Finely grated zest of 1 lemon
1/2 teaspoon freshly squeezed lemon juice, plus more to taste
Freshly ground black pepper to taste
1/4 cup chopped salted pistachios
Grated Parmesan cheese, for serving (optional)

1. In a food processor fitted with a fine grating attachment, shred the squash. (Or use a box grater, but it will be harder to do. You could also just cut it into small cubes; it won't dissolve into a sauce but will be differently pleasing.) In a small saucepan, bring the stock to a simmer. Melt the butter in a large skillet over medium heat. Add the leeks and cook, stirring them occasionally, until they are soft, 5 to 7 minutes. Stir in the garlic and cook it until fragrant, about 1 minute. Add the rice, squash, rosemary, and salt. Stir until most of the grains of rice appear semitranslucent, 3 to 4 minutes. This means they have absorbed some of the fat from the pan, which will help keep the grains separate from each other as they form their creamy sauce.

2. Pour the wine into the pan and let it cook off for about 2 minutes. Add a ladleful of stock (about 1/2 cup) and cook, stirring it constantly and making sure to scrape around the sides, until most of the liquid has evaporated.

Continue adding stock, a ladleful at a time, and stirring almost constantly until the risotto has turned creamy and thick, and the grains of rice are tender with a bit of bite, 25 to 30 minutes (you may not need all the stock). Pluck out the rosemary branch and stir in the lemon zest, lemon juice, and black pepper. Taste and add more salt and lemon juice if needed. Garnish with the pistachios and optional cheese before serving.

What Else?

- Risotto is one of those things you might think is difficult to make, which is completely untrue. It's no harder than oatmeal, though you do have to stir the pot with some regularity. I write in the recipe that you should stir it almost constantly, which is what I do. During most of its cooking time, I'm there at the stove, stirring away. But I do take a few short breaks to perhaps chop up some pistachios or pour myself a glass of seltzer. As long as the breaks are very short, they won't compromise your risotto; just make sure to resume stirring with gusto and make sure to stir around the edges of the pan.

- Sometimes, when I'm feeling lazy, I skip the step of putting the stock in a small saucepan over low heat next to my risotto pot, then ladling it a little at a time. The idea behind that technique is that you don't want to bring the temperature of the risotto pan down too much as you add the stock, so adding small amounts of boiling (or at least steaming) stock works best. To cheat, sometimes I'll pour the stock into a glass measuring cup, then stick it in the microwave for a few minutes to heat it up. Then I'll pour it directly from the measuring cup into the pan, a few splashes at a time. As it cools, I'll just stick it back in the microwave to reheat it. I find this easier than the pot-and-ladle method (especially since my measuring cups are dishwasher safe and my pots are not). You can do it either way.

- I've also heard tell that in restaurants, which are generally too busy for all that ladling and stirring, they add all the stock at the beginning and let the

[CONTINUED]

risotto bubble gently until finished, giving it a quick stir every so often. This technique might be worth a try if you are seriously opposed to the stirring process, though I'd try it first on a night when I'm not expecting company or feeding a hungry marathoner.

- I've made the cheese optional because I do leave it out for Daniel and he loves the risotto without it. However, I like to shower my portion with good Parmesan.

FARRO PASTA WITH SPICY SALAMI TOMATO SAUCE AND FRESH MINT

This is what Daniel ate the night before he ran his second New York City marathon. Pasta is the traditional premarathon meal, and as much as I wanted to honor that tradition, I have to admit that I was also craving the stuff. I love pasta even though I've never run more than five consecutive miles in a row.

Daniel and I both prefer whole wheat pasta for most of our meals at home, though we do break out the white stuff every once in a while. For a premarathon meal, my instinct would have been to cook up the simple white carb, but Daniel asked for whole grains. It might not be as efficient a carb to digest, but it would stay with him longer, he said, which was a plus.

I was able to score some really good nutty farro pasta at my local gourmet market. Whole wheat would have worked nicely, too, but I like the slightly more rustic texture and earthier flavor of the farro stuff.

Since the farro pasta was my starting point, I knew it would be best served topped with a hearty, spicy, assertively flavored sauce that would stand up to its full flavor.

Daniel requested something without a lot of meat, so I nixed a bolognese.

Instead, I made a sauce inspired by Franny's, my neighborhood Italian restaurant. There, Andrew Feinberg, the chef (and my friend), makes a fiery salami pasta rich with plum tomatoes and good, herby olive oil. For his version, he makes his own extra-spicy sopressata for the sauce. I used regular spicy sopressata fired up with a good pinch of crushed red pepper flakes.

Andrew tops his pasta with plenty of grated cheese, but I left it off and added some chopped fresh mint instead.

Daniel and I gobbled it up, and it gave him the energy he needed to rock the race and me enough to cheer him on from the sidelines in the most energetic fashion I could muster.

¼ cup extra-virgin olive oil

½ yellow onion, chopped

1 garlic clove, thinly sliced

½ teaspoon kosher salt, plus additional to taste

Pinch freshly ground black pepper, plus additional to taste

1 (28-ounce) can San Marzano tomatoes

FOR THE PASTA

1 pound dry farro or whole wheat pasta of a short thick shape,
    such as penne

½ pound spicy sopressata, casing removed

2 tablespoons extra-virgin olive oil, plus additional
    for serving

½ teaspoon dried Sicilian pepper or red pepper flakes

Chopped fresh mint, for garnish

1. To make the tomato sauce, heat the oil in a medium saucepan over medium-low heat. Add the onion, garlic, ½ teaspoon salt, and a small pinch of black pepper. Cook, covered, until the vegetables are very soft, 5 to 7 minutes. Pour in the tomatoes and their liquid. Continue to simmer until the sauce thickens and the oil separates and rises to the surface of the sauce, about 25 minutes. Run the sauce through a food mill fitted with the large disc; season with additional salt and pepper.

2. To make the pasta, bring a large pot of heavily salted water to a boil. Cook the pasta until very al dente (remove it about 2 minutes before al dente). Drain the pasta well.

3. Cut the sopressata into batons about 2 inches long and ¼ inch thick.

4. In a large, straight-sided skillet, heat the oil over medium-high heat. Add the sopressata and cook, stirring occasionally, until the sausage is light golden and has rendered some of its fat. Pour in the tomato sauce and Sicilian pepper or red pepper flakes. Cook over high heat until the sauce looks dry and turns golden around the edges, about 8 minutes.

5. Remove the sauce from the heat and stir in 1/4 cup water. Add the pasta. Return the skillet to the heat and cook, tossing occasionally, until the sauce reduces and tightens around the pasta, 2 to 3 minutes.

6. Divide the pasta among individual serving plates. Drizzle each plate with olive oil, sprinkle with mint, and serve.

What Else?

- Farro pasta is a nutty, chewy whole grain pasta made from farro, an ancient form of wheat. If you can't get your hands on some, use any whole grain pasta, so long as it is a sturdy, tubular-shaped pasta that mimics the size of the salami. A ribbed or corkscrew-shaped pasta works, too. The sauce will cling to its textured surface and little bits will get stuck, in a good way, in the crevices. Because of this, slippery spaghetti or linguine are not the right pasta choices for this dish.

- If you don't want to use sopressata, you can substitute another salami, so long as it is meaty and spicy with a soft texture. Pepperoni makes a great alternative. Make sure your butcher cuts it into thick chunks versus slices so you can cut it into batons.

- The tomato sauce is a good, basic recipe that you can use on anything calling out for tomato sauce. We keep small containers of it in the freezer and defrost them to top whole wheat macaroni for Dahlia's supper. It makes giving her a homemade meal as quick as boxed mac and cheese, and so far, she likes it even better. (I have no illusions that this will persist.)

- At Franny's, Andrew uses Pecorino Romano to top this pasta. I left it off when I made this for Daniel. But speaking of cheese, when I heated up leftovers for lunch, I added a few dollops of fresh ricotta and it was superb. The mild milky soft cheese mitigated the hot peppers and made everything very creamy.

GARLICKY BROCCOLI RABE

Hearty pasta and risotto dishes need bright, zesty, green vegetable side dishes to wake up all that sleepy, starchy comfort food. Sautéed bitter broccoli rabe is one of my favorites. It's simple, very tasty, and I make it all the time in the colder months. That's when all the best crucifers are in season, and when I tend to crave the deep, sharp flavor of bitter greens tamed with plenty of garlic and chile.

Sometimes, when I'm home alone and not in the mood for a full-on meal (maybe I've had a big restaurant lunch or ate too many cookies in the afternoon), I'll make this for dinner and serve it on its own. It's so satisfying that I don't miss the pasta or polenta or chicken or whatever usually goes with it. And one large, fluffy bunch of broccoli rabe perfectly feeds one (this one, anyway) for a spunky solo dinner.

2 tablespoons extra-virgin olive oil

2 fat garlic cloves, finely chopped

Large pinch red pepper flakes

1 large bunch broccoli rabe, tough stems removed

3/4 teaspoon kosher salt

Serves 1 or 2

Heat the oil over medium heat until hot. Add the garlic and pepper flakes; cook until fragrant, about 30 seconds. Add the broccoli rabe and salt and toss well. Cook 1 minute. Stir in 2 tablespoons water. Cover the pan and cook until tender, 3 to 4 minutes. If necessary, cook, uncovered, to evaporate any excess water in the pan.

What Else?

- The trinity of oil, garlic, and red pepper flakes is one I turn to a lot on nights when we want a quick side dish. Some nights it's broccoli rabe, others I do regular broccoli, broccolini, kale, or fresh spinach. It's such a great combination I'm sure it would make my shoe taste good, though I have no intention of trying that.

- I've seen many recipes that call for blanching the broccoli rabe before sautéing it. I've never found that necessary. Covering the pan after sautéing it will steam-cook it without the need for another pot to wash, because, really, who wants to deal with more dishes?

- This could easily be stretched into a meal. Brown some sausage in the pan before adding the garlic and broccoli rabe, then toss in some pasta at the end. You might add an extra drizzle of oil and some grated Parmesan to bring the whole mixture together.

SPICY THREE-MEAT CHILI

Daniel's favorite dish is chili. Whenever I ask him what he wants for dinner, chili is nearly always the answer, no matter the season. So I make chili all year long. I make it in the winter, when it's frigid and foul. I make it in the spring, when it's rainy and raw. I even make it in the summer on the hottest, steamiest days. But autumn seems to me to be the ideal chili-cooking time of year, when the weather is cold enough to warrant long, savory simmering, and you still might be able to snag the last of the bell peppers or jalapeños at the farmers' market.

Whenever I whip up a potful, Daniel will gladly eat the whole thing in a matter of days, one heaping portion after another, unless I stash a few containers in the freezer first.

Daniel is a chili enthusiast of the most democratic ilk. He likes beef and bean chilis as much as turkey chilis, vegetarian chilis, beanless, Texas-style chilis, even tofu chilis. As long as it's stewy, spicy, and filled with lots of little tasty tidbits to munch, he will finish the bowl and lick the spoon.

I'm a lot pickier when it comes to chili. I try my hardest to avoid situations where I am forced, out of politeness, to consume vegetarian chili, tofu chili, or chili made from anything with wings.

Give me hoof meat and spice, and beans and vegetables if you like, and I'll be happy.

This chili satisfies us both. I like the trio of meats, which gives it a complex, interesting flavor—sweet from the veal, brawny from the pork, and robust from the beef, and we both like the combination of fresh chiles and dried chili powder, and all the vegetables and beans for textural amusement.

The odd man out, so to speak, is Dahlia, who, as of now, doesn't like chili at all. We assume one day that will change, and until then, she'll have plenty of opportunities to try the dish again and again, year in and year out.

Serves 8

1 tablespoon extra-virgin olive oil
1 pound ground beef or bison

2$\frac{1}{2}$ teaspoons kosher salt, plus additional to taste

1$\frac{1}{2}$ teaspoons freshly ground black pepper, more to taste

1 pound ground pork

1 pound ground veal

1$\frac{1}{2}$ tablespoons tomato paste

1 medium green bell pepper, seeded and diced

1 medium red bell pepper, seeded and diced

1 medium onion, finely chopped

2 garlic cloves, finely chopped

1 to 2 jalapeños, seeded and finely chopped, to taste

3 tablespoons chili powder, plus additional to taste

1 (28-ounce) can crushed tomatoes

1 (28-ounce) can whole peeled tomatoes, broken up
with a fork

3 cups cooked kidney beans or 2 (15 ounce) cans,
drained and rinsed

Chopped fresh cilantro, for serving

Lime wedges, for serving

1. Heat the oil in a large pot over medium-high heat. Add the beef and cook, breaking up with a fork, until well browned, 5 to 7 minutes. Season the meat with $\frac{1}{2}$ teaspoon each salt and pepper. Remove the beef with a slotted spoon and transfer the meat to a paper towel–lined platter. Repeat the cooking process twice more with the pork and veal. Season each with $\frac{1}{2}$ teaspoon salt.

2. Add the tomato paste to the pot. Cook, stirring, until the paste is golden brown, 1 to 2 minutes. Stir in the peppers, onion, garlic, and jalapeño. Cook until the vegetables are softened, 7 to 10 minutes. Stir in the chili powder and a pinch of salt; cook 1 minute. Add the tomatoes, beans, 2 cups water, and the remaining salt. Return the meat to the pot. Reduce the heat to medium and simmer for 30 minutes.

3. Ladle the chili into bowls. Sprinkle with cilantro and serve with lime wedges.

What Else?

- Don't underestimate the power of good-quality chili powder. I usually use a mix of mild and hot New Mexico chili powders, but there are so many kinds to choose from, from mild anchos to super-spicy chile de arbol, and since the art of serious chili making is really all about achieving that perfect blend, you should feel free to experiment. If you want to go whole hog, you can even buy dried whole chiles and grind your own in a spice grinder.

- I love finishing my food with garnishes, which is another reason to love chili. Fresh garnishes like chopped herbs, scallions, tomato, or avocado are a great contrast to the slow-simmering flavor of chili and, on my bowl at least, a dollop of sour cream.

- If you get to the bottom of your chili leftovers and want to stretch them to feed your whole family one more time, stir in some cooked elbow macaroni or rinsed, canned hominy.

- If possible, buy your ground veal at your farmers' market instead of the supermarket. You can read why on page 241. If you really can't do veal, then just do half pork and half beef, or all pork or all beef, or even turkey if you like. As long as you've got 3 pounds of ground meat of some type, the recipe will come out fine.

- This freezes well and I always try to have a container in the freezer. It makes Daniel happy to know that the chili is there when he wants it.

- Daniel likes chili over brown rice, either coconut or plain (page 49). I like it best with corn bread (page 333).

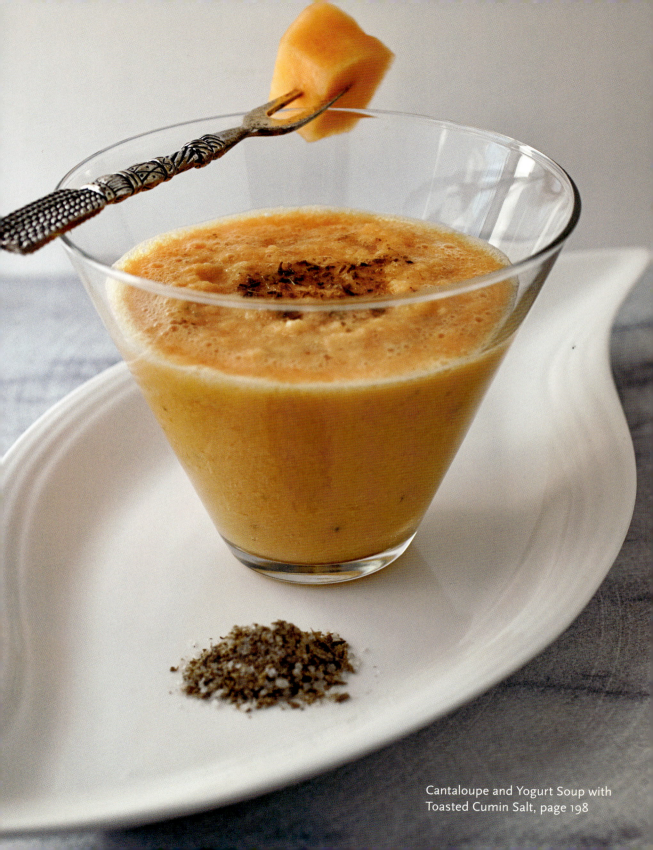

Cantaloupe and Yogurt Soup with
Toasted Cumin Salt, page 198

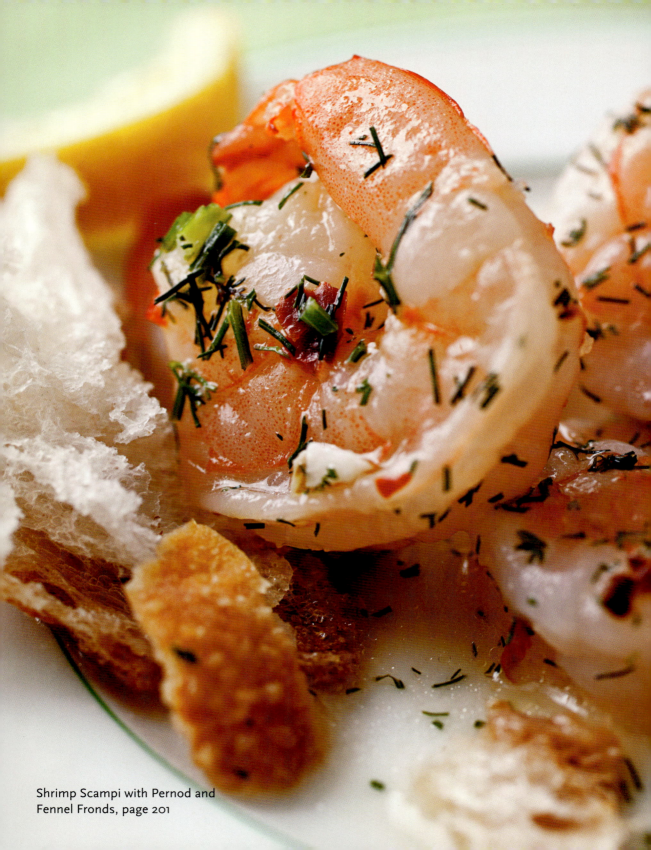

Shrimp Scampi with Pernod and
Fennel Fronds, page 201

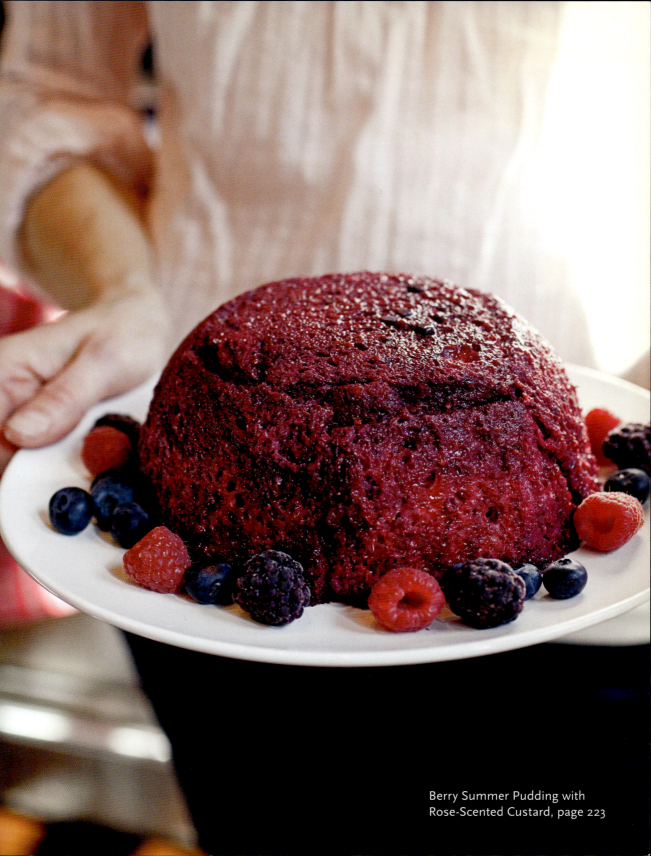

Berry Summer Pudding with
Rose-Scented Custard, page 223

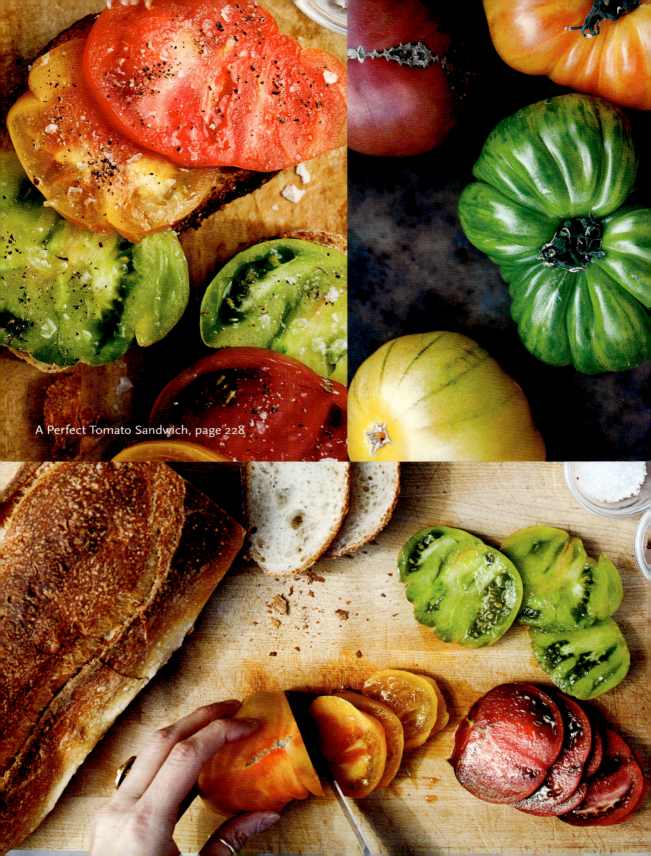

A Perfect Tomato Sandwich, page 228

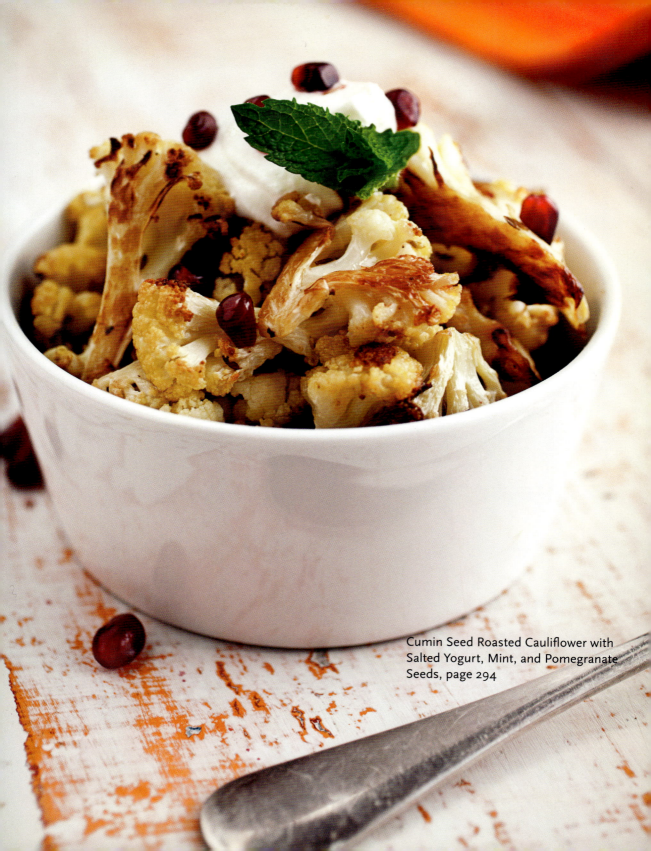

Cumin Seed Roasted Cauliflower with Salted Yogurt, Mint, and Pomegranate Seeds, page 294

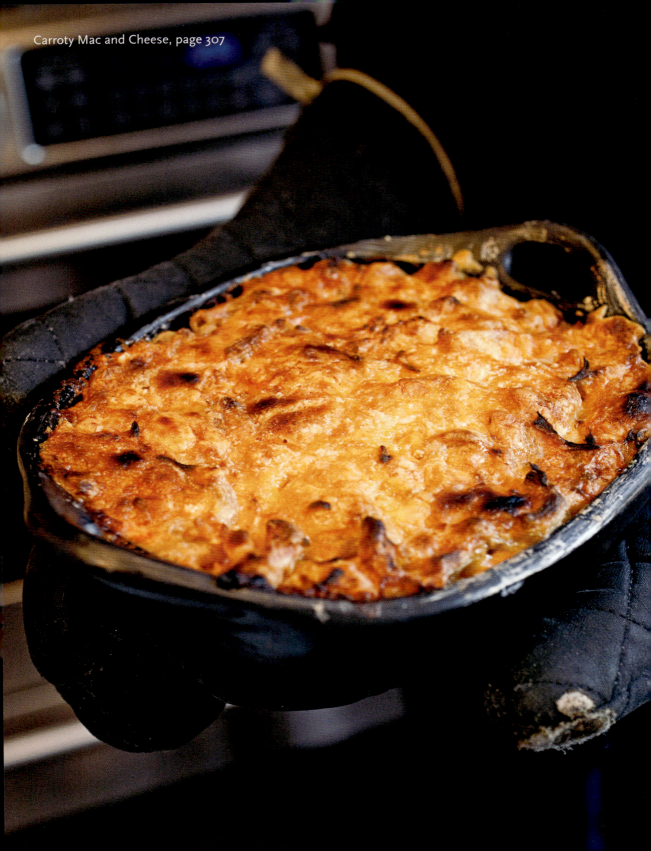

Carroty Mac and Cheese, page 307

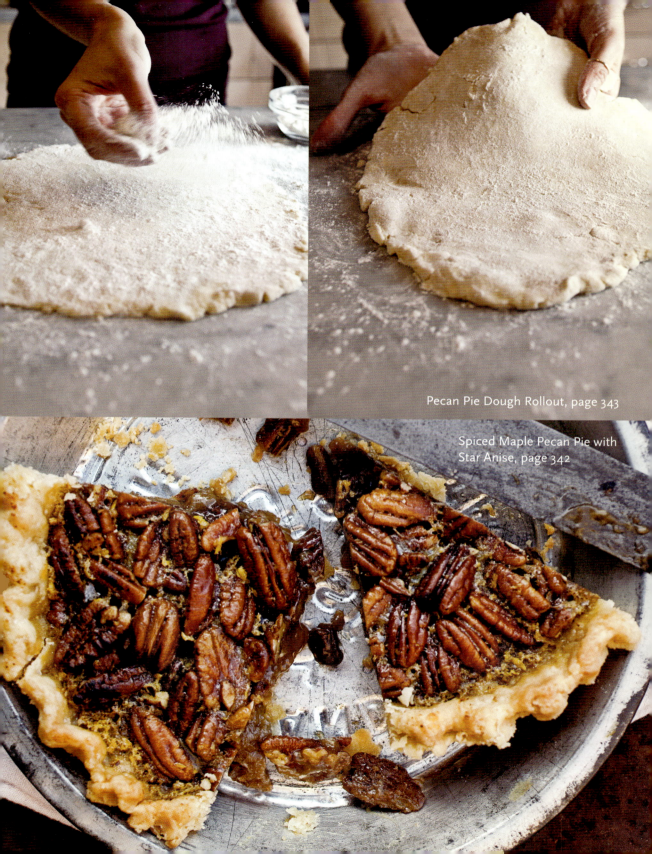

Pecan Pie Dough Rollout, page 343

Spiced Maple Pecan Pie with Star Anise, page 342

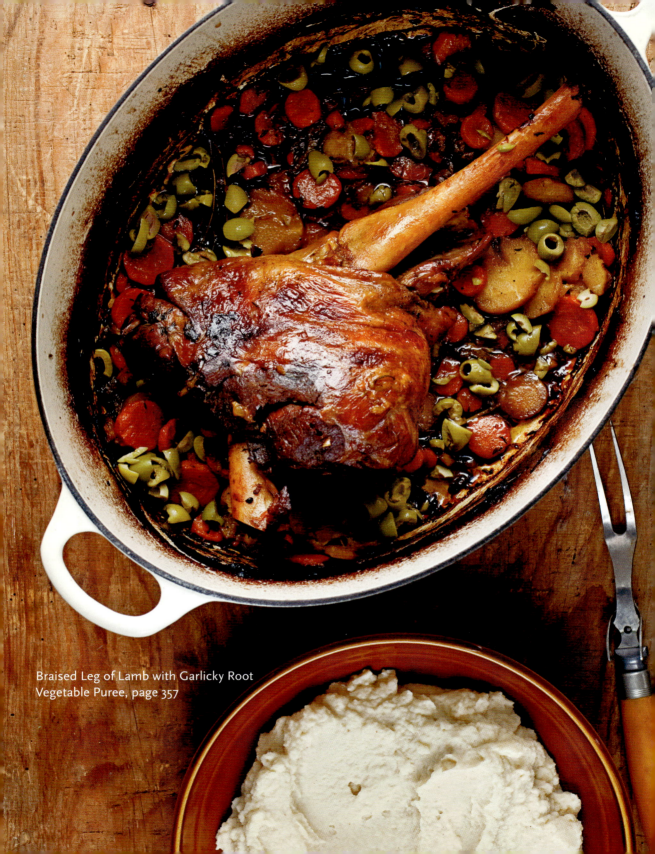

Braised Leg of Lamb with Garlicky Root
Vegetable Puree, page 357

HONEY WHOLE WHEAT CORN BREAD

I think corn bread is the perfect thing to serve with chili, especially this fluffy, honeyed, very buttery corn bread, which crumbles easily into your chili bowl and contrasts sweetly with the fiery stew.

Like every corn bread I've ever met, this one is best served warm from the oven, slathered with butter and more honey. But unlike some of its brethren, it's moist enough to serve at room temperature, or perhaps toasted if you've got any left over, which we never seem to.

The whole wheat flour isn't really in-your-face detectable here. I think it adds a pleasing, earthy, toasty nuance. And of course it increases the fiber count ever so slightly, from practically none to just a little. But if you don't have any on hand, just substitute all-purpose flour. No one but you will know the difference.

Makes 1
(9-inch round) loaf

Serves 6

1 cup yellow cornmeal

1/3 cup whole wheat flour

1/3 cup all-purpose flour

1 tablespoon baking powder

1 1/2 teaspoons kosher salt

1 cup sour cream

1/2 cup whole milk

1/3 cup honey

2 large eggs

1/4 teaspoon baking soda

8 tablespoons (1 stick) unsalted butter

1. Preheat the oven to 375°F.
2. In a large bowl, whisk together the cornmeal, flours, baking powder, and salt. In a separate bowl, whisk together the sour cream, milk, honey, eggs,

[CONTINUED]

and baking soda. Gently fold the wet ingredients into the dry ones until just combined.

3. Place a 9-inch cast-iron skillet (see What Else?) over high heat until hot. Melt the butter in the skillet, swirling the pan to coat the bottom and sides with butter. Pour the butter into the batter and stir to combine. Scrape the batter into the skillet.

4. Bake until the top is golden and a toothpick inserted into the center comes out clean, 25 to 30 minutes.

What Else?

- Cast iron is terrific for corn bread making because it gets nice and hot, which helps the corn bread form a crisp, golden bottom crust. But if you haven't got a cast-iron skillet (and, really, they are cheap enough so you should), you can melt the butter in the microwave and use a 9-inch-square pan for baking instead.

- I set out to make a corn bread that was wholesome but light, which is what I got. But if you want to adjust the proportion of whole wheat to all-purpose flour to make the corn bread heartier, you can swap out all of the all-purpose flour.

- Chili powder, chopped fresh thyme leaves, fresh corn kernels, sliced scallions, or a handful of grated cheese would all make nice additions to this corn bread. You can stir any extras right into the batter.

SHREDDED BRUSSELS SPROUTS WITH PANCETTA AND CARAWAY

For years, my preferred way to eat Brussels sprouts was halved and roasted until the outer leaves got crisp and dark brown, while the centers softened and mellowed. The recipe was almost too easy. I just tossed the halved sprouts with olive oil and salt, and roasted them at high heat until they were blistered and black-edged, and then ate them by the bowlful.

Then recently I met a whole other kind of Brussels sprouts dish at my parents' house, and I liked it a lot. Instead of cut in halves, these sprouts were shredded, then quickly sautéed over high heat so the edges turned golden. Compared to the halved sprouts there was more browning, which meant more caramelization and a sweeter flavor. But another thing I liked was the way the shreds absorbed all the good seasonings in the pan, which never quite penetrate the dense halved sprouts in the same way.

The shredded sprouts that my parents made were suffused with Indian spices—mustard seed, cumin, and coconut—and they were delicious. But I wanted to take the dish in another direction when I made it a few weeks later, and that was toward Europe, so I could use plenty of fatty pork products to crisp in the pan and render out fat to coat the shreds.

I meant to use bacon, but in the end decided on pancetta, which isn't smoked and has a gentler, porkier flavor that I hoped would bring out the sweetness of the sprouts.

I also added a pinch of caraway seeds to the pan because the pile of shredded sprouts in my food processor looked a little like green cabbage, and green cabbage reminds me of Germany, and Germany reminds me of caraway.

It was a long, circuitous road to get to the pan of vegetables, but the sprouts were pure bliss—tender, crisp-edged, pork-coated, and garlicky—and well worth the journey.

1 pound Brussels sprouts

3 tablespoons extra-virgin olive oil

4 garlic cloves, finely chopped

1½ teaspoons caraway seeds

4 ounces pancetta, diced small (½ cup)

½ teaspoon kosher salt

Freshly ground black pepper to taste

1. Use a paring knife to trim the bottoms of the sprouts; peel away any browned leaves. In a food processor fitted with the slicing blade, shred the Brussels sprouts. Toss the sprouts with 2 tablespoons oil, the garlic, and the caraway seeds.

2. Heat the remaining 1 tablespoon oil in a large skillet over medium-high heat. Add the pancetta and cook until golden, 3 to 5 minutes. Add the Brussels sprouts mixture and cook, tossing, until wilted, 1 to 2 minutes. Season with the salt and pepper.

What Else?

- If you don't have a food processor with a slicing blade, you can cut the Brussels sprouts in quarters and just sauté them for a few extra minutes. (Cover the pan for a few minutes to help them steam as they sauté.) Or you can use a knife, but it will take a while.

- You really do just want to cook the Brussels sprouts until they are wilted, since the texture is best when the sprouts still have a bit of crunch. In fact, I sometimes eat a salad variation of this dish where I don't cook the sprouts at all, so don't worry about undercooking them.

- This is a great dinner party side dish. Guests love it, it's pretty all-purpose (pairing well with beef, chicken, or fish), and you can shred the sprouts the day before without any problem. Just store them in the fridge in a resealable plastic bag or airtight container.

ROASTED ACORN SQUASH, HONEY, SMOKED PAPRIKA, AND SAGE SALT

Seasoned salts are all the rage, and these days it's a rare gourmet market that doesn't proudly display a shelf of the wildly conceived crystals, made from all manner of herbs, spices, and even nuts and meats.

I've even been lured into purchasing some of them. But I can never seem to remember to use them, and they usually sit, unloved and untouched, in my cabinet until I finally throw them out.

Not so this woodsy-flavored sage salt. One day, faced with a surplus of sage from the pot on the deck, which needed to get used before it succumbed to a hard winter freeze, I made up a batch. Instead of banishing it to the nether regions of the spice drawer, I left it on the counter in a little bowl, then proceeded to sprinkle it on anything that needed a touch of salt.

And in my kitchen, that's a lot of things. I used it on eggs, I used it on soups, I used it on chili (page 330) and on salads.

But the best dish I made with the salt was hands down this simple roasted acorn squash, which I also tossed with honey and smoked paprika for depth and sweetness. It would make a great Thanksgiving side dish if you doubled or tripled the recipe, and it's just as good at room temperature as it is hot (important if you're making it for Thanksgiving).

And if you don't want to make the sage salt yourself, you could probably even top the squash with one of those purchased salt blends you've probably been tempted into buying. It happens to the best of us.

Serves 4 to 6

2 medium acorn squash, trimmed
2 tablespoons extra-virgin olive oil
2 teaspoons honey
1 teaspoon smoked sweet paprika

[CONTINUED]

½ teaspoon kosher salt

4 large sage sprigs (about 16 nice leaves)

2 teaspoons coarse sea salt

1. Preheat the oven to 350°F. Slice the squash crosswise into ½-inch rings. Use a spoon to scoop the seeds from the center of each ring; discard or reserve for toasting (see What Else?).

2. In a small bowl, whisk together the oil, honey, paprika, and kosher salt. Arrange the squash on a large baking sheet; pour the paprika oil over the squash and toss well to combine. Place the sage leaves in a small baking pan.

3. Transfer both pans to the oven. Roast the sage leaves until just crisp, about 10 minutes; transfer to a rack to cool. Raise the heat to 400°F. Continue roasting the squash, turning once, until tender and light golden, 20 to 25 minutes more.

4. Transfer the squash to a platter. Crumble the sage in a small bowl (you should have about 1½ teaspoons) with the coarse salt; sprinkle some of the sage salt over the squash and serve.

What Else?

- If you want to toast your own squash seeds, rinse the seeds and let dry in a single layer on paper towels (it's okay if a few bits of squash pulp cling to the seeds). Toss with oil and salt and toast in a 350°F oven until crisp and golden, 12 to 15 minutes.

- You don't have to use acorn squash for this recipe. Any sliced squash will take to the seasonings. I really like it with delicata and sweet dumpling squash, too.

- You only need a little bit of sage salt for this recipe, and leftovers will be wonderful on all kinds of foodstuffs. I can report that it is especially tasty as a garnish for white bean stew or sprinkled over slices of hot buttered whole grain toast. But use it with an open hand and you won't be disappointed.

STICKY CRANBERRY GINGERBREAD

There is ginger cake, and there is gingerbread. And although the terms are often used interchangeably, to me, the two desserts are as different as chocolate and vanilla.

The way I see it, ginger cake is refined and elegant. It's mild-mannered, smooth, tender, and delicate, breaking apart into large fluffy crumbs as soon as it meets the knife. Ginger cake willingly accepts a frosting (preferably of the cream cheese variety) and is not out of place at a wedding or fancy party.

Gingerbread is ruder, wetter, and stickier. In fact, other than a pungent, spicy-ginger flavor, stickiness is probably gingerbread's most distinguishing characteristic. And when I say sticky, I mean, a glossy, tacky surface that's practically oozing honey or molasses or whatever syrupy substance is holding the cake crumb together. If it doesn't have the sticky outer layer, it might as well be cake.

I'm happy to report that after much tinkering, this gingerbread recipe is sticky through and through, thanks to the inclusion of several dollops of homemade cranberry compote, which fall to the bottom of the pan, then caramelize and nearly candy in the oven. It gives the cake a toffee-like texture, and also adds a tart, bright cranberry flavor, which melds nicely with the ginger.

Once you've got your ginger confections sorted out, you'll never confuse this with cake. And you might like it even better.

Serves 8 to 10

2 cups fresh or frozen cranberries (1/2 pound)

1 cup granulated sugar

1/2 cup (1 stick) unsalted butter

2/3 cup dark brown sugar

1/2 cup whole milk

1/2 cup molasses

[CONTINUED]

1/4 cup golden syrup

1 1/2 cups all-purpose flour

1 tablespoon ground ginger

1/2 teaspoon ground cinnamon

1/2 teaspoon baking powder

1/2 teaspoon kosher salt

1/4 teaspoon baking soda

1/4 teaspoon freshly ground black pepper

2 large eggs, lightly beaten

1 tablespoon grated fresh gingerroot

1. Preheat the oven to 350°F and line a 9-inch-square baking pan with parchment.

2. In a small, heavy-bottomed saucepan, stir together the cranberries, granulated sugar, and 1 tablespoon water. Stir the cranberries over medium heat until the sugar is completely dissolved and the cranberries form a sauce that is syrupy and bubbling thickly, about 10 minutes. Aim to have about half of the cranberries broken down, with the remainder more or less whole.

3. In a separate saucepan, stir together the butter, brown sugar, milk, molasses, and golden syrup over medium heat. Bring it to just barely a simmer and then remove it from the heat. Do not let it come to a boil, or the mixture might curdle.

4. In a large bowl, sift together the flour, ginger, cinnamon, baking powder, salt, baking soda, and black pepper. Beat in the butter-molasses mixture and then beat in the eggs. Stir in the ginger.

5. Scrape the batter into the pan. Drop fat dollops of cranberry sauce onto the surface of the cake batter. Drag a long, slender knife through the batter in a swirly design, as if you are marbling a cake. Transfer the cake to the oven and bake until the top is firm and a toothpick inserted in the center comes out clean, about 50 minutes. Transfer the pan to a wire baking rack and let the cake cool completely before eating it.

What Else?

- You might notice that your beautifully swirled crimson cranberries sink to the bottom of the pan. This is okay, even good—as the cake bakes, they will form this delicious, chewy, caramelized cranberry bottom crust on the cake.

- Make sure to grease the pan really well. It is a sticky cake, after all.

- This cake will get you through an entire day. I eat it for breakfast, with my afternoon mug of tea, and I even serve it for dessert to dinner guests (sometimes that just means Daniel and Dahlia).

- If you're making it for a special occasion that requires getting out your dessert plates, you might also consider adding a bourbon-spiked dollop of whipped cream.

SPICED MAPLE PECAN PIE
WITH STAR ANISE

I never thought to simmer down maple syrup until it turns thick, viscous, and extremely maple-y until I made Bill Yosses's maple ice cream recipe. Yosses, the pastry chef at the White House and a good friend of mine (we wrote a cookbook together), reduces the syrup to eliminate as much of the water as possible, which gives the smoothest, silkiest textured ice cream imaginable, with an intense maple flavor. He also recommends reducing maple syrup for any recipe in which you want an extremely vibrant maple character.

After trying his amazing ice cream recipe, I began to think about what else might benefit from reduced maple syrup's profound caramel sweetness, and came up with pecan pie.

The problem with most maple pecan pies is that the maple becomes shy and quiet in the company of all those assertive toasted nuts. Simmering down the syrup, I hoped, would help it hold its own.

So I tried it and it worked beautifully, with the sweet maple in perfect balance with the nutty pecans. It became my go-to pecan pie technique for years.

Then one Thanksgiving, I decided to add a layer of complexity to the pie by infusing whole spices into the maple syrup while it was simmering. I chose star anise because I thought the sharp, woodsy fennel flavor would add an unexpected nuance to the classic combination of maple and nuts.

That's just what happened. My pie was warm and licorice-y from the anise, toasty from the roasted pecans, and as syrupy, sugary, and toothachingly sweet as a proper pecan pie should be. I wouldn't have it any other way, though a dollop of crème fraîche tempers the gooey filling without compromising its integrity.

Makes 1 (9-inch) pie
_____

Serves 8

FOR THE PIECRUST

1¹/₄ cups all-purpose flour

¹/₄ teaspoon salt

10 tablespoons unsalted butter, chilled and cut into ¹/₂-inch pieces

2 to 5 tablespoons ice water

FOR THE FILLING

1 cup maple syrup

¹/₂ cup Demerara or raw sugar

8 whole star anise

2 cups pecan halves

3 large eggs

4 tablespoons (¹/₂ stick) unsalted butter, melted

2 tablespoons dark aged rum

¹/₄ teaspoon kosher salt

Whipped crème fraîche, for serving

1. To make the crust, in a food processor, briefly pulse together the flour and salt. Add the butter and pulse until the mixture forms lima bean–size pieces (three to five 1-second pulses). Add ice water 1 tablespoon at a time, and pulse until the mixture is just moist enough to hold together. Form the dough into a ball, wrap with plastic, and flatten into a disc. Refrigerate at least 1 hour before rolling out and baking (or up to a week, or freeze for up to 4 months).

2. On a lightly floured surface, roll out the piecrust to a 12-inch circle. Transfer the crust to a 9-inch pie plate. Fold over any excess dough, then crimp as decoratively as you can manage.

3. Prick the crust all over with a fork. Freeze the crust for 15 minutes or refrigerate for 30 minutes. Preheat the oven to 400°F. Cover the pie with aluminum foil and fill with pie weights (you can use pennies, rice, or dried beans for this; I use pennies). Bake for 20 minutes; remove the foil and weights and bake until pale golden, about 5 minutes more. Cool on a rack until needed.

[CONTINUED]

4. To make the filling, in a medium saucepan over medium-high heat, bring the maple syrup, sugar, and star anise to a boil. Reduce to a simmer and cook until the mixture is very thick, all the sugar has dissolved, and the syrup measures 1 cup, 15 to 20 minutes. Remove from the heat and let sit for 1 hour for the anise to infuse.

5. While the syrup is infusing, toast the nuts. Preheat the oven to 325°F. Spread the pecans out on a baking sheet and toast them in the oven until they start to smell nutty, about 12 minutes. Transfer to a wire rack to cool.

6. Remove the star anise from the syrup. Warm the syrup if necessary to make it pourable but not hot (you can pop it in the microwave for a few seconds if you've moved it to a measuring cup). In a medium bowl, whisk together the syrup, eggs, melted butter, rum, and salt. Fold in the pecan halves. Pour the filling into the crust and transfer to a rimmed baking sheet. Bake until the pie is firm to the touch but jiggles slightly when moved, 35 to 40 minutes. Let cool to room temperature before serving with whipped crème fraîche.

What Else?

• If you can get Grade B maple syrup, which has a fuller, richer flavor than the usual Grade A stuff, your pie will be even more maple-y. That's what I use.

• Toasted cashews would be a really nice, buttery, soft substitute for the pecans.

• If you want to skip the star anise, go right ahead. You'll be left with a stellar, simpler, and more traditional pie with an excellent, deep maple flavor.

• Sometimes I like to drizzle melted extra-bitter (72 percent) chocolate all over the top of the pie. It helps cut the sweetness and adds chocolate, which never hurts anything.

DECEMBER

CORNMEAL BLINI WITH SALMON CAVIAR

Every holiday season, I always find an excuse to make these luxurious corn-meal blinis with crème fraîche and caviar. Whether I'm having a full-fledged holiday party, or a small Christmas Eve dinner for a few friends, I'll fry up a batch of the tiny, buttery, grainy pancakes, top them with crème fraîche and the best caviar I can afford in a given year, and serve them with Champagne. I don't think there's anything more festive to kick off a celebratory meal.

Makes 36 blinis

1 cup fine cornmeal

1 cup all-purpose flour

½ teaspoon baking soda

1 teaspoon baking powder

1 teaspoon kosher salt

1 tablespoon sugar

3 large eggs, lightly beaten

1 cup buttermilk or plain yogurt

1 cup milk

4 tablespoons (½ stick) unsalted butter, melted

Olive oil, for frying

2 cups crème fraîche

Salmon roe or other caviar, for topping

Snipped chives, for topping

1. Preheat the oven to 250°F.
2. In a medium bowl, combine the cornmeal, flour, baking soda, baking pow-der, salt, and sugar and stir well to mix. Add the eggs, buttermilk or yogurt, milk, and melted butter, and mix until smooth.
3. Heat a frying pan over medium heat until hot, then brush with oil. Using a spoon and working in small batches, drop tablespoons of batter into the

pan. When bubbles form evenly on the top of the blini, turn (just once) and cook until golden.

4. Transfer the first batch of cooked blini to a heatproof plate lined with paper towels and keep warm, covered, in the oven. Repeat with the remaining batter.

5. To serve, top each warm blini with a dollop of crème fraîche, a smaller dollop of salmon caviar, and a sprinkling of chives. Serve immediately.

What Else?

- If you want to turn this into more traditional blini, you can substitute buckwheat flour for the cornmeal. I have done them both ways many times and slightly prefer the cornmeal because I like its sweet butteriness, which I think melds better with the salty caviar, compared with the deep earthiness of the buckwheat blini.

- Caviar isn't everyone's bag (or everyone's budget). Fortunately, the world is full of delicious blini-topping alternatives. Some of my favorites include smoked salmon, fresh ricotta and honey, crumbled blue cheese and chives, and Greek yogurt and pomegranate seeds.

- This batter keeps pretty well, so feel free to stir it together in the morning for a party that evening. Or save leftover blini batter to make into cornmeal pancakes for breakfast the next day. Just keep the batter covered and refrigerated.

- Sour cream or Greek yogurt can be substituted for the crème fraîche if you can't find it. Or, if you plan ahead, you can make your own. In a jar with a lid, mix a tablespoon of buttermilk or plain yogurt with a cup of heavy cream. Leave it in a warm spot, shaking the jar occasionally, until the mixture is thicker and sour tasting, 24 to 36 hours (it will get more sour as it sits, so when it tastes sour enough for you, it's ready). Then put the jar in the fridge, where it will continue to thicken as it chills. If it's still runny when you want to serve it, whisk it until it thickens. I usually have to do this to make it thick enough to top blinis without running everywhere.

BEET AND CABBAGE BORSCHT WITH DILL

There are elaborate, hearty, meaty borschts that take all day to make and require myriad ingredients. And then there are simple, vegetable-based borschts that celebrate the purity of sweet beets and cabbage without many other distractions. This is a borscht of the latter type. It's brothy, light, and full of soft, shredded cabbage along with tender bits of magenta beet, which turn the broth bright red, or fuchsia pink if you swirl in a mound of sour cream at the end.

This is just the kind of soup to make during the busy holiday season because it's quick, tasty, festive on account of its exuberant color, and also very, very good for you with all those vegetables bobbing in the bowl.

The recipe is based on one that I thought I got from Patricia Wells's *Food Lover's Guide to Paris*. When I lived there in my junior year abroad, her book was my bible, and I roamed around the city trying to hit as many of the places she listed as I could—at least the cafés and wine bars and pastry shops, which were my priorities.

The recipe that I remember called for using cooked beets, which are easily available in Paris, where most beets are sold already roasted. I made the soup while I was living there, using purchased cooked beets, and then continued to make the soup back home in New York, roasting my beets first before adding them to the broth.

At some point, I got lazy and stopped roasting the beets. I simply shredded them up and tossed them into the soup pot with the cabbage, and I can't say I missed whatever layer of flavor I'd always assumed the roasting contributed. The soup was, as it always had been, ruby colored and sweetly flavored, with a tang from a touch of red wine vinegar and green freshness from chopped dill.

I was curious about what Patricia Wells had to say about the roasted beets in her recipe, but when I went back to find it in my latest edition of her book, I couldn't. It had either been recently expunged, or I'm getting things all mixed up about where I got the recipe in the first place. In any case, this is my version, a tribute to an excellent original, whatever its source.

Serves 4 to 6

½ small head green or red cabbage, cut into quarters and cored
4 medium raw beets, peeled and quartered
4 tablespoons (½ stick) unsalted butter
1 medium onion, peeled and finely chopped
2 fat garlic cloves, finely chopped
6 cups chicken or vegetable broth
1¾ teaspoons kosher salt
¾ cup chopped fresh dill
1½ teaspoons red wine vinegar
Sour cream or Greek yogurt, for serving

1. Pass the cabbage through the feed tube of a food processor fitted with the coarse grating blade. Transfer the grated cabbage to a large bowl. Pass the beets through the feed tube and add the grated beets to the bowl with the cabbage.
2. Heat the butter in a large pot over medium heat until the foam subsides. Add the onion. Cook, stirring, until the onion is slightly softened, about 5 minutes. Add the garlic; cook 1 minute. Add the cabbage and beets. Increase the heat to medium-high and cook, tossing occasionally, until the cabbage is wilted, about 10 minutes.
3. Add the broth and 1 teaspoon salt to the pot. Bring the liquid to a boil. Reduce the heat to medium-low and simmer gently, uncovered, for 30 minutes. Stir in the dill, remaining ¾ teaspoon salt, and vinegar. Ladle the soup into bowls and serve, topped with a dollop of sour cream.

What Else?

- Sometimes I add coriander seeds to this soup. I toast them first in a dry skillet, then lightly crush them before adding them to the pot. They add a haunting, musky flavor that I love.

- I'm crazy about beets, but the eternal problem with them is that it's tough to know how sweet they are going to be until you are eating them. If your beets are really sweet, you might need to add a splash more vinegar to the soup, less if yours are on the earthy side.

- If a soup comprised of mostly cabbage and beets doesn't sound substantial enough to you, you can bulk it out by adding some diced potatoes along with the cabbage.

- Once, when I was at my parents' house for lunch, my mother served borscht topped with tzatziki, a Greek dip made from yogurt, garlic, chopped dill, and diced cucumber. It was wonderful, and ever since I'll sometimes do the same if I can get nice cucumbers. And even if I can't, mixing some minced garlic, a pinch of salt, and a handful of dill into the sour cream before dolloping it into the bowl is most refreshing and delightful.

GOLDEN PARSNIP LATKES

Shredded parsnip makes these crispy pancakes sweeter than the usual potato latkes, and the parsnips' dry flesh renders them extraordinarily crunchy, too.

I came up with the recipe during a brief period of parsnip experimentation, after I brought home a huge bag of the pale roots without any kind of plan about how to use them. Some found their way into a comforting, pureed soup (page 56), some I roasted simply with olive oil and salt, and the remainder got shredded and fried into latkes during one of the nights of Hanukkah, though I can't remember which. I do remember Daniel's and Dahlia's reaction to the brittle-textured, sweet-and-salty morsels. Not that they said much; they were too busy chewing. But gobbling speaks louder than words.

Makes about 18 latkes

1 pound parsnips (about 3 medium), peeled and cut in half crosswise
1 medium onion, peeled and cut into quarters
1/2 cup all-purpose flour
2 large eggs
2 1/2 teaspoons kosher salt
1 teaspoon baking powder
1/2 teaspoon freshly ground black pepper
Chicken fat, duck fat, or olive oil, for frying

1. Using a food processor with a coarse grating disc, grate the parsnips and onion. Transfer the mixture to a clean dish towel and squeeze and wring out as much of the liquid as possible.
2. Working quickly, transfer the mixture to a large bowl. Add the flour, eggs, salt, baking powder, and pepper and mix until the flour is absorbed.
3. In a medium heavy-bottomed pan over medium-high heat, pour in about 1/4 inch of oil. Once the oil is hot (a drop of batter placed in the pan should sizzle), use a heaping tablespoon to drop the batter into the hot pan, cooking 3 to 4 latkes at one time. Use a spatula to flatten and shape the drops into

[CONTINUED]

discs. When the edges of the latkes are brown and crispy, 2 to 3 minutes, flip. Cook until the second side is deeply browned, another 2 to 3 minutes. Transfer the latkes to a paper towel–lined plate to drain. Repeat with the remaining batter.

What Else?

- You can garnish these with all the usual potato pancake toppers, including sour cream and applesauce, but they are also wonderful plain, sprinkled with a little more salt.

- Serve these with any stewed, braised meats, including the pot-roasted lamb on page 103, or the braised oxtails on page 25. Or if you're roasting a chicken, these would make an unexpected and tasty side dish.

- When you make latkes, expect your kitchen to get a little smoky and grease splattered. So wear an apron, open the windows if it's not too cold to do so, and crank up the fan.

A Dish by Another Name

- To make regular Crispy Potato Latkes, just substitute potatoes for the parsnips.

SAUTÉED BAY SCALLOPS WITH ROSEMARY, CAPERS, AND ISRAELI COUSCOUS

Tiny wild bay scallops are as sweet as candy, and when I can get the freshly caught, opalescent little critters, I'll sometimes eat them like ocean-flavored gumdrops, straight out of hand, one after the other.

Usually, though, I cook them lightly before consuming, and this is one of my all-time favorite ways to showcase the pillowy mollusks.

The recipe starts out pretty predictably. I sauté the scallops in butter with plenty of garlic, wine, lemon, and a pinch of crushed red pepper flakes, similar to shrimp scampi. Then I shake things up by stirring a spoonful of capers and some cooked beads of Israeli couscous into the pan. The capers add a welcome sharp tang to the sweet scallops while the couscous pearls roll around the tongue like bursting bubbles, exploding with buttery, garlicky flavors.

The dish's effervescent personality always makes me want to serve it with a glass of sparkling wine, or at least a little seltzer with a squeeze of lemon. Given that wild bay scallops come into season right around the holiday festivities, you can guess which bottle I reach for.

Serves 2 to 3

1 cup dry Israeli couscous

2 rosemary branches

3 tablespoons unsalted butter

2 garlic cloves, finely chopped

Pinch red pepper flakes

1/2 cup dry white wine

1 pound bay scallops, patted dry

1 tablespoon drained capers

1/2 teaspoon kosher salt, plus additional to taste

[CONTINUED]

1 teaspoon freshly squeezed lemon juice
¼ cup chopped fresh parsley

1. Bring a pot of salted water to a boil. Add the couscous and cook 3 minutes; drain.
2. Using the flat side of a knife, lightly bruise the leaves of the rosemary branches (I put the rosemary under the knife, then lean on it). Melt the butter in a large skillet over medium heat. Add the garlic, rosemary, and red pepper flakes. Cook, stirring, for 1 minute.
3. Pour in the wine and increase the heat to medium-high. Simmer until the liquid has reduced by half, about 2 minutes. Stir in the couscous, scallops, capers, and salt. Cook, stirring, until the scallops are just cooked through, 2 to 3 minutes. Stir in the lemon juice and parsley; serve.

What Else?

- Farmed bay scallops, while not quite as intensely saline as the wild ones, are a very sustainable, inexpensive, and perfectly lovely substitute.

- Shrimp also work well here, and they're very pretty, too, with their bright pink color against the capers' deep green.

- A bay leaf or a few thyme sprigs can stand in for the rosemary branch. If you can find lemon thyme, it's especially nice with the scallops.

- I like to use whole wheat Israeli couscous, which is sometimes labeled "pasta pearls." Fregola, which is pasta pearls that have been toasted, also work beautifully in this dish, though I've yet to see whole wheat fregola, so if you see a package in a specialty shop, assume they are made from semolina.

WINTER SALAD WITH FENNEL, RADICCHIO, WALNUTS, AND MANCHEGO

When the weather turns cold and all the tender salad greens start to look as if they've seen better days, I know I can always reach for radicchio and it won't let me down.

With the bright-hued look of an overgrown Christmas tree ornament, the tightly coiled magenta leaves unfurl once sliced, expanding and blossoming onto the cutting board in a florid heap.

One snowball-size head will fill a salad bowl for four, especially when it's augmented with some thinly sliced fennel and garnished with crunchy nuts and salty, creamy cheese, as I've done here. It's a filling salad that makes a fine lunch on its own. Or serve it as the first course to an elegant dinner, of which I hope you'll enjoy many during this jovial time of year.

Serves 4

1 1/2 tablespoons freshly squeezed lemon juice
1/2 teaspoon kosher salt
1/2 teaspoon freshly ground black pepper
1 fat garlic clove, finely chopped
1/4 cup extra-virgin olive oil
1/4 pound aged manchego or Parmesan cheese
1/3 cup toasted walnuts, finely chopped
1 large head radicchio, quartered lengthwise and cored
1 large fennel bulb, fronds chopped and reserved

1. In a bowl, whisk together the lemon juice, salt, pepper, and garlic. Whisk in the oil. Use a Microplane or other grater to finely grate 2 ounces of the cheese (you'll get about 1/2 cup). Whisk the grated cheese and walnuts into the vinaigrette (it should be fairly thick).

[CONTINUED]

2. Thinly slice each radicchio wedge crosswise and transfer to a large salad bowl. Trim the stems from the fennel and remove the outer layers. Cut the fennel bulb in half from top to bottom. Using a mandoline or very sharp knife, shave the fennel into paper-thin slices. Add to the salad bowl.

3. Pour the vinaigrette over the salad and toss well. Use a vegetable peeler to shave the remaining 2 ounces of cheese into curls. Toss into the salad. Taste and adjust any seasonings, if necessary.

What Else?

- If you can get nice salad greens, you can add them here and it will look spectacularly pretty. Just make a double batch of the vinaigrette and toss the whole thing with whatever nice, flavorful greens you've managed to snap up, such as arugula, watercress, or baby spinach.

- Radicchio is a bitter lettuce. I find that the sweetness of the fennel is enough to temper it for my taste, but you can add a handful of raisins or chopped dates if you find you need more.

- Instead of fennel, sometimes I like to add some orange or pink grapefruit segments to the bowl. It makes a bolder, juicier salad that works really nicely with roasted meats and chicken.

- If you can't get radicchio or don't like it, you can substitute 2 or 3 Belgium endives. It makes a beautifully pale salad with a delicate, sweet character.

BRAISED LEG OF LAMB WITH GARLICKY ROOT VEGETABLE PUREE

Maybe it's because I grew up spending Christmas Eve in Chinatown with my clan of New York City Jews, but celebrating the holiday has always felt like a work in progress. Since I'm not wedded to any one particular tradition, I've jumped around, trying different ones on for size.

When I was married to an Italian-American man, he and I made elaborate feasts of seven fish for Christmas Eve, just like his family always did, and served them to a group of close friends.

After our divorce, I invited the same friends over for the holiday but cooked up whatever festive party food I felt like making; though I have to admit that I took fish off the menu.

Then Daniel moved in and we started from scratch, looking to create new holiday traditions together.

One of them has become braising a large hunk of meat. For our family, it's the ideal holiday dish. We can braise it in advance, serve it to friends on Christmas Eve, then reheat the leftovers for Christmas dinner, when we are too tired from opening presents and our annual Christmas walk around the park (one of my new favorite traditions) to want to cook anything new.

We've varied the contents of the braising pot over the years, but keep coming back to leg of lamb because we both love it, and since we don't eat it very often, it seems like a special meal. Plus braising a bone-in leg of lamb is an excellent way to cook it. The marrow flows into the sauce, thickening and seasoning it, while the meat collapses and becomes spoonably soft.

In this recipe, I've added anchovy and olives to the pot to give the sauce a tangy depth that works well with all the rich meat. It's especially nice served over a smooth, sweet root vegetable puree spiked with garlic, which acts like a velvety sauce. On Christmas Day, we toss the leftovers with pasta. It's a wonderful new two-day tradition, boiled down into one pot.

1 shank end leg of lamb (4½ pounds), bone in, rinsed and patted dry

3 tablespoons olive oil

1 tablespoon plus ½ teaspoon kosher salt

1¾ teaspoons freshly ground black pepper

2 cups chicken stock

1 (750-ml) bottle fruity white wine

3 small onions (¾ pound), peeled, halved, and thinly sliced

3 large carrots (¾ pound), peeled and sliced into ½-inch rounds

1 large parsnip (¼ pound), peeled and sliced into ½-inch rounds

4 anchovy fillets

2 rosemary sprigs

2 sage or thyme sprigs

1 bay leaf

½ cup pitted and coarsely chopped green olives

2 garlic cloves, finely chopped

FOR THE GARLICKY ROOT VEGETABLE PUREE

1 large celeriac bulb, peeled and diced

2 medium Yukon Gold potatoes, diced

2 large parsnips, peeled and diced

4 garlic cloves, peeled

2 bay leaves

2 tablespoons plus 1 teaspoon kosher salt, more to taste

8 tablespoons (1 stick) unsalted butter, to taste

Freshly grated nutmeg to taste

1. To prepare the lamb: Preheat the oven to 450°F. Rub the lamb with 1 tablespoon oil, and season it with 1 tablespoon salt and 1½ teaspoons black pepper.

2. In a medium saucepan over medium-high heat, bring the stock and wine to a boil; allow it to bubble gently and reduce while you sauté the vegetables, about 10 minutes or so.

3. In a large Dutch oven over medium-high heat, warm the remaining 2 tablespoons oil. Add the onions and cook, stirring occasionally, until soft, 7 to

10 minutes. Stir in the carrots and parsnip, anchovies, 1/4 teaspoon salt, the remaining 1/4 teaspoon pepper, rosemary, sage, and bay leaf. Turn off the heat and pour in just enough of the stock-wine mixture to cover the vegetables. Place the lamb, fatty-side up, on top of the vegetables.

4. Transfer the pot to the oven and cook, uncovered, for 25 minutes. Then add the remaining stock, cover the pot, and reduce the heat to 325°F. Cook for 1 1/2 hours, at a bare simmer, reducing the heat if necessary, then turn the lamb over. Cook 1 1/2 hours longer and turn the lamb over again. Uncover the pot and stir in the olives. Cook another hour, turning the lamb after 30 minutes. At this point the lamb should be soft enough to cut with a serving spoon. If not, cover the pot and continue to cook until it is.

5. To prepare the root vegetable puree, in a large saucepan, combine the celery root, potatoes, parsnips, peeled garlic cloves, and bay leaves. Pour in 12 cups water and 2 tablespoons kosher salt. Over medium-high heat, bring to a boil; reduce the heat and simmer until tender, 20 to 25 minutes. Drain, discard the bay leaves, and transfer the root vegetables and garlic to a food processor. Add the butter, remaining teaspoon salt, and nutmeg; process until very smooth. Taste and add more salt if necessary. Keep warm or reheat before serving.

6. Just before serving, mash the finely chopped garlic and the remaining 1/4 teaspoon salt to form a paste. Stir it into the lamb's pan juices.

7. To serve, make a bed of root vegetable puree on each plate. Cut the lamb with a serving spoon, and lay some of it over the puree, along with some vegetables and pan juices.

What Else?

- Lamb legs can be really big. Sometimes they are so big that they barely fit into your pot and the bone sticks out in a very ungainly manner. If you think of it while you are at the butcher, ask them to trim the bone end down a bit, which will make for less awkward handling.

[CONTINUED]

- If you make the braise the day before you want to serve it, you'll be able to degrease the pot. Let the lamb cool, then chill overnight (if it's cold out, I will often just put the whole covered cast-iron pot on my deck). In the morning, spoon off the layer of yellow fat that's risen to the surface and discard it. Then reheat the braise before serving. Do this before adding the garlic paste, which should be done just before serving.

- Shanks can be substituted for the leg of lamb if you like. You'll need 6 of them. If you like, you can brown them before braising. I usually do because it does intensify the lamb-y flavor, and unlike trying to brown an unwieldy bone-in leg of lamb, browning shanks is easy. Then the shanks will cook in about $2\frac{1}{2}$ to 3 hours.

ROASTED RUTABAGAS WITH MAPLE SYRUP AND CHILE

Every time I roast a rutabaga, I mentally thank Bill Maxwell of Maxwell Farms. He was the one who suggested, then cajoled, then finally insisted that I try rutabagas again when I hadn't had one in years.

"They're so sweet, I don't know why people aren't going crazy for them," he said, motioning to a milk crate brimming with the waxy vegetables.

"Because they're hard to cut, and then when you cook them, they don't taste like anything," I said.

"Those must have been old and overgrown. Just try one of these and tell me what you think," he said, pressing a pineapple-size specimen into my hands.

Bill suggested I boil it, mash it, and serve it with caramelized onions.

I went home and roasted it instead. I'd read online that roasted rutabaga was the ideal way to cook the vegetable, caramelizing its juices and enhancing its sweetness.

And Bill was right: The rutabaga was wonderful—soft, mellow, browned around the edges, and tasting a little like roasted butternut squash with a pleasantly sharp, turnipy edge.

Since that day, I roast rutabagas all the time, often glazed with a little maple syrup or honey to help deepen the browning. In this recipe, I've added a pinch of chile for a spicy kick, but the rutabaga is good without it, too, and perhaps more appropriate if you're feeding small children.

The one thing I haven't done yet is to try Bill's recipe for a rutabaga mash. But I will soon, now that his rutabaga authority has been so firmly established.

[CONTINUED]

1½ pounds rutabagas, peeled and cut into ¾-inch cubes

2 tablespoons extra-virgin olive oil

1 tablespoon maple syrup

¾ teaspoon kosher salt

⅛ teaspoon cayenne

1. Preheat the oven to 400°F.
2. In a large bowl, combine the rutabagas, oil, maple syrup, salt, and cayenne; toss well to combine. Spread the rutabagas in a single layer on a large baking sheet. Roast, tossing occasionally, until the rutabagas are tender and dark golden, about 40 minutes.

What Else?

- Like turnips, rutabagas can be an acquired taste. If you're still getting used to it, you can substitute some of the rutabagas with potatoes, carrots, parsnips, or whatever other root vegetables you are into at the moment.

- If you haven't worked with rutabagas before, they are a little bit more watery than most root vegetables. I think this gives them a refreshing feel, even when roasted, but it does mean that you probably won't achieve that totally crisp, dark brown crust you usually get on roasted vegetables. A nice golden hue is just about right. The maple syrup will also help caramelize them a bit.

RED CHARD WITH
PINE NUTS, GARLIC, AND
GOLDEN RUM RAISINS

This is one of those serendipitous dishes, a combination of ingredients that I wouldn't have ever thought to put together myself; but once I tasted the dish, it seemed inevitable.

It happened one Christmas Eve, when Daniel and I had a dinner party that was larger than usual, and I asked a friend of a friend, Amber Campion, to come and help me with the cooking and cleanup.

To tell the truth, although I'd planned most of the menu ahead, there were a few dishes I figured I'd improvise at the last minute, including a side dish of red chard.

I bought several nice bunches, cleaned them, and put them next to the stove, figuring I'd sauté them with garlic and chile flakes.

But with the party in full swing, I was too distracted to return to the stove, and Amber offered to sauté them with pine nuts and raisins, one of her favorite dishes. It sounded good to me.

Left on her own, Amber rooted through the cupboards and found a little container of golden raisins, so she threw them into the sauté pan.

The chard was so remarkably good that everyone asked Amber for the recipe, including me.

She explained what she did, and it sounded simple enough—but too simple for the nuanced flavors on our plates. There had to be some secret ingredient in that chard, and I got a little ticked off that she wasn't divulging it.

Finally, I realized what it was: aged dark rum. Amber had accidentally added a container of rum raisins I had made for some holiday baking but had never used. The rum added a mild smokiness and sweetness, which set off the slightly bitter chard to perfection. Now, even if I don't add raisins, I'll often splash a little dark rum into a pan of sautéed greens. It's my secret ingredient.

3/4 cup golden raisins

1/4 cup dark rum

4 large bunches red chard

2/3 cup pine nuts

1/3 cup extra-virgin olive oil

2 large garlic cloves, finely chopped

3/4 teaspoon kosher salt

1/4 teaspoon freshly ground black pepper

1. In a small saucepan, combine the raisins, rum, and 2 tablespoons water. Simmer over medium-low heat until the raisins are plump and most of the liquid has evaporated, about 3 minutes.

2. Remove the center ribs from the chard and discard. Slice the leaves 1 inch thick. In your largest skillet over medium heat, toast the pine nuts, tossing occasionally, until golden, about 5 minutes. Transfer the nuts to a bowl. Heat the oil in the pan over medium-high heat. Add the garlic and cook, stirring, until fragrant, about 30 seconds. Add the chard, a handful at a time, cooking until wilted, 6 to 8 minutes total. Season the greens with the salt and pepper. Stir the raisins and nuts into the skillet; toss to combine.

What Else?

- The rum is not essential in this recipe, but it does give the dish a boost of sweetness, depth, and complexity. You can use white wine, orange juice, or water instead.

- You can make this with almost any green including spinach, broccoli rabe, and kale. Just remember that the thicker and hardier the green, the longer it will take to cook, so you may have to add a few minutes to the cooking time. If the pan dries out, add a few tablespoons of water.

- Slivered almonds are a good pine nut stand-in.

SWEET AND SPICY CANDIED NUTS

These fragrant, glossy candied nuts make the perfect holiday gift when scooped into a pretty glass jar and tied with a silky, bright ribbon.

I made a batch one December, intending to do just that. But the batch was small, and by the time I'd "tasted" enough of them to make sure they were worthy of all my dearest friends, there were hardly any left. Instead, I put the remainders in a glass bowl on the table next to the Christmas Eve eggnog and let everyone snack on them while imbibing. The crunchy, candied nuts were a huge hit, gone in minutes with people asking for more. Alas, there weren't any.

But next year, I'm going to make a double batch and give them out to everyone I know. Or perhaps I should make that a triple.

Makes 5 cups

1 cup light brown sugar
1 large egg white
1 pound mixed nuts
1 teaspoon kosher salt
$\frac{1}{2}$ teaspoon ground cinnamon
$\frac{1}{2}$ teaspoon freshly grated nutmeg
Large pinch cayenne
Pinch ground cloves

1. Preheat the oven to 300°F. Line a baking sheet with parchment.
2. In a large bowl, whisk together the sugar and egg white. Add the nuts and toss to combine. In a separate bowl, stir together the salt, cinnamon, nutmeg, cayenne, and cloves. Sprinkle the mixture over the nuts and toss well.
3. Spread the nuts in a single layer on the prepared baking sheet. Bake, tossing occasionally, until the nuts are fragrant and almost dry to the touch, about 30 minutes.

What Else?

- I used mixed nuts because I had a motley collection of nuts left over from other baking projects, but you could always make sweet and spicy candied cashews or sweet and spicy candied pecans instead.

- These nuts can be used for so much more than snacking: They would be delicious in a salad of bitter greens with a nice tart vinaigrette. You could layer them with sliced fruit and yogurt for a breakfast parfait. You can chop them up and use them to garnish cakes. I have even sprinkled them over roasted root vegetables and baked sweet potatoes.

- But if you are using them for snacking and are among pork lovers, crumble in some bacon. It provides an incredible smoky, savory element that is completely addictive.

SPEEDY COCONUT EGGNOG

There is nothing I don't like about eggnog. It's rich, it's creamy, it's fluffy and frothy. It is, for me, the pinnacle of wintertime tippling. But for my dairy-eschewing husband? Not so much.

One winter, right when the weather started to turn snowy, I was experimenting with a butterscotch Scotch eggnog recipe for my column in the *New York Times* when I felt a little sorry for Daniel, who was sipping a decidedly unexciting bourbon on the rocks. So I concocted this dairy-free nog for him using unsweetened coconut milk, which is my favorite dairy replacer.

It tastes like a version of a coquito (a Puerto Rican nog that uses Coco Lopez), only much less sweet. And it's nearly as fluffy, frothy, and festive as a traditional nog—only even better, because this one we can share.

Serves 2, but can be scaled up or down

2 large eggs
3/4 cup unsweetened coconut milk
1 tablespoon sugar, or to taste
1 shot rum or bourbon
1 shot brandy
Freshly grated nutmeg, for garnish

> Place the eggs, coconut milk, sugar, rum or bourbon, and brandy in a blender and puree until smooth. Serve garnished with lots of nutmeg and with an ice cube, if you like your nog a little chilly.

What Else?

- For a foamier, fuller-bodied nog, separate the eggs. Blend the yolks with the rest of the ingredients. Whip the whites with a few tablespoons sugar until soft peaks form and fold into the nog. Serve with nutmeg and a spoon.

- Adjust the booziness of this nog to suit the tastes of your fellow imbibers.

A Dish by Another Name

- For a more traditional Holiday Eggnog, substitute whole milk or half-and-half for the coconut milk. If you like a sweeter nog, add another pinch or two of sugar.

Bonus Recipes

FROM MELISSA CLARK'S COOKBOOK

In the Kitchen with A Good Appetite

Whether dining at a restaurant or eating at home, my parents had a rule that my sister and I actually followed when we were growing up: Try everything once and if you don't like it, you don't have to try it again.

If we refused, punishment was subtle but palpable parental disappointment.

My sister, less susceptible to that kind of guilt trip, was a pickier eater and all-around more normal child when it came to food.

"Eww!" she'd exclaim over a piece of stinky Vacherin.

I was more afraid of losing my parents' esteem than slipping down a raw oyster or licking a wobbly cube of foie gras aspic. The upside was that most of those things actually tasted good, and it was thrilling, even at age nine, to suck the unctuous marrow-prize out of a craggy veal bone.

Flash-forward to my putative adulthood. Now, when it comes to home cooking, I am just as intrepid.

After all, if there's one thing I learned from my parents, it's that getting lost is all part of finding a great meal. For me these days, this means cooking without recipes, and creating dishes from my cravings coupled with what's available in the supermarket, seasoned with the mishmash of food memories I've amassed over the decades.

With work and family life ever present, my recent recipes tend to be on the quicker, more straightforward side of gourmet, but no less delectable for that. And every one has a story behind it, stories that I explored in my last book, *In the Kitchen with A Good Appetite*.

And here, I am offering a selection of recipes from that book that are dear to my heart. I hope they become dear to yours, too.

Crème Brûlée French Toast
with Orange Blossom Water

1 cup packed light brown sugar

8 tablespoons (1 stick) unsalted butter, melted and still warm

2 large eggs, well beaten

1½ cups milk

2 tablespoons freshly squeezed orange juice

2 teaspoons orange blossom (flower) water

1 teaspoon vanilla extract

½ teaspoon ground cinnamon

¼ teaspoon kosher salt

1 (10-ounce) French baguette, sliced diagonally, 1 inch thick (about 20 slices)

Time: 35 minutes

Serves 4 to 6

1. Preheat the oven to 375°F. In a medium bowl, whisk together the brown sugar and butter until the sugar is completely dissolved. Pour the mixture into a large rimmed baking sheet (about 11 × 17 inches).

2. In a pie pan or other shallow dish, combine the eggs, milk, orange juice, orange blossom water, vanilla, cinnamon, and salt. Coat both sides of the bread slices in the egg mixture, letting the bread soak up the custard for at least 15 minutes, then place them on the prepared baking sheet over the brown sugar mixture. Bake for 25 to 30 minutes, or until the tops of the bread are golden brown and the sugar is bubbling.

3. Serve immediately while still hot, with the crunchy brown sugar side up, spooning more of the pan syrup over the tops.

NOTE: To oven-bake your bacon at the same time, place strips of bacon on another large rimmed baking pan (about 11 × 17 inches) and place it in the oven on the rack below the toast (so none of the bacon grease accidentally splatters on the toast). The bacon will cook in about the same time as the toast (25 minutes or so), though watch it carefully. When it's done to taste, take it out of the oven and drain the strips on a brown paper bag or paper towels. If you like it sweet, you can drizzle a little maple syrup over the bacon before baking.

Pan-Roasted Asparagus with Fried Eggs and Anchovy Bread Crumbs

Time: 10 minutes

Serves 2
as an appetizer
or side dish

3 tablespoons extra-virgin olive oil

3 tablespoons unseasoned, preferably homemade bread crumbs

1 anchovy fillet, minced

1 small garlic clove, minced

Kosher salt to taste

1/4 teaspoon freshly grated lemon zest

1 bunch asparagus, trimmed

Pinch freshly ground black pepper

2 large eggs

1. Heat 1 tablespoon of the oil in a large skillet over medium heat. Add the bread crumbs and anchovy and cook, stirring occasionally, until the bread crumbs are browned and toasted, about 2 minutes. Stir in the garlic and a large pinch of salt and sauté until fragrant, 1 to 2 minutes longer. Add the lemon zest, then transfer the mixture to a small bowl.
2. Wipe out the skillet with a paper towel and return it to the heat. Add another tablespoon of the oil and then add the asparagus and a pinch of salt and pepper. Cover and cook, stirring and shaking the pan occasionally, until the asparagus is tender, 5 to 6 minutes. Transfer the asparagus to a serving plate and sprinkle with the bread crumb mixture.
3. Add the remaining tablespoon of the oil to the skillet and return it to the heat. Crack in the eggs and fry until just set but still runny, 2 to 3 minutes. Slide the eggs on top of the asparagus and serve.

Roasted Eggplant with Basil Green Goddess Dressing

1 large eggplant (about 1 pound), scrubbed, trimmed, and cut into
    1-inch cubes

5 tablespoons extra-virgin olive oil

1¼ teaspoons kosher salt

¼ cup crème fraîche or sour cream

2 tablespoons mayonnaise

2 anchovy fillets, chopped

2 garlic cloves, chopped

1 tablespoon chopped fresh chives

1 tablespoon chopped fresh parsley

1 tablespoon chopped fresh basil

1½ teaspoons freshly squeezed lemon juice

¼ teaspoon freshly ground black pepper

Time: 30 minutes

Serves 4

1. Preheat the oven to 400°F. In a rimmed baking sheet, toss the eggplant with the oil and ¾ teaspoon kosher salt. Arrange the cubes in a single layer and roast for 30 minutes, stirring once or twice.

2. While the eggplant is roasting, make the dressing. In the bowl of a food processor, place the crème fraîche or sour cream, mayonnaise, anchovies, garlic, chives, parsley, basil, lemon juice, pepper, and the remaining ½ teaspoon salt. Run the motor until the mixture is fully combined and bright green. Serve the dressing alongside or drizzled over the eggplant.

Shrimp for a Small Kitchen (Shrimp with Capers, Lemon, and Feta)

Time: 10 minutes

Serves 2 to 3

2 tablespoons extra-virgin olive oil

3 garlic cloves, minced

1 pound large shrimp, shelled and cleaned

1/3 cup crumbled feta

Juice of 1/2 lemon

1 to 2 tablespoons capers to taste

Kosher salt and freshly ground pepper to taste

2 tablespoons chopped fresh cilantro or basil, plus additional for garnish

1. Heat the olive oil in a large skillet over medium heat. Add the garlic, stirring, and cook until fragrant but not browned, about 1 minute. Stir in the shrimp, then add the feta, lemon juice, capers, and salt and pepper.
2. Continue stirring over the heat until the shrimp become just opaque and the sauce begins to thicken, about 2 minutes. Add the cilantro or basil and stir to combine. Serve garnished with additional herbs, if desired.

My Mother's Garlic and Thyme–Roasted Chicken Parts with Mustard Croutons

Time: 1 hour and 10 minutes

Serves 4

Country bread, ciabatta, or other sturdy bread, preferably stale, sliced 1/2 inch thick

Mustard, as needed

Extra-virgin olive oil, as needed

1 1/2 teaspoons kosher salt, more as needed

1/2 teaspoon freshly ground black pepper, more as needed

1 (4- to 5-pound) chicken, cut into 8 serving pieces, rinsed and patted dry

1 head garlic, separated into cloves

1 bay leaf, torn into pieces

1/2 bunch thyme sprigs

[CONTINUED]

1. Preheat the oven to 425°F. Lay the bread slices in the bottom of a heavy-duty roasting pan in one layer. Brush with mustard, drizzle liberally with olive oil, and sprinkle with salt and pepper.
2. Season the chicken all over with salt and pepper and place the pieces on the bread, arranging the white meat in the center and the dark meat and wings around the sides. Scatter the garlic cloves, bay leaf, and thyme over the chicken and drizzle everything with more oil (take care to drizzle the garlic cloves).
3. Roast the chicken until it's lightly browned and the thigh juices run clear when pricked with a knife, about 50 minutes. If you like, you can crisp the skin by running the pan under the broiler for a minute, though you might want to rescue the garlic cloves before you do so they don't burn (if you don't plan to eat them, it doesn't matter so much). Serve the chicken with pieces of the bread from the pan.

Quick-Braised Chicken with Moroccan Spices, Lemon, and Olives

1 lemon, ends trimmed (see Note)

1 tablespoon plus 1½ teaspoons kosher salt

3 pounds chicken thighs and drumsticks, rinsed and patted dry

1½ teaspoons freshly ground black pepper

3 to 4 tablespoons extra-virgin olive oil

1 large onion, chopped (about 1½ cups)

1 fat garlic clove, minced

1 teaspoon grated fresh gingerroot

1 tablespoon ground coriander

1 tablespoon ground cumin

1½ teaspoons sweet paprika

½ teaspoon ground turmeric

½ teaspoon ground cayenne

2 to 3 cups chicken stock

¼ teaspoon crumbled saffron

Time: 1 hour

Serves 3 to 4

½ cup good-quality green olives, pitted if desired (I used pitted picholines)

3 tablespoons dried currants or diced dried apricots (optional)

2 tablespoons chopped fresh cilantro or mint

1. Thinly slice the lemon crosswise into rounds. Cut the rounds into quarters. Place the lemon in a small saucepan with water just to cover and stir in 1 tablespoon kosher salt. Bring the mixture to a boil, then reduce the heat and simmer for 5 minutes. Drain well and rinse the lemon under cold water.

2. Season the chicken with the remaining 1½ teaspoons kosher salt and the pepper. In a large, deep skillet, heat 3 tablespoons of the oil over medium-high heat. Place the chicken in an even layer in the skillet (do this in batches, if necessary) and brown on both sides, about 10 minutes. Transfer the chicken to a paper towel–lined plate to drain.

3. If the skillet looks dry, add the remaining tablespoon of oil. Add the onion and sauté until soft, about 5 minutes. Stir in the garlic, ginger, coriander, cumin, paprika, turmeric, and cayenne, and cook for 1 minute more.

4. Add the chicken and stir to coat with the spice mixture. Pour the stock into the skillet until two-thirds of the chicken is covered. Stir in the saffron and bring to a boil. Reduce the heat to medium-low, cover, and let simmer for about 25 minutes.

5. Uncover and add the lemon slices, olives, and dried fruit, if desired, stirring to combine. Cover and return to a simmer until the chicken is cooked through, about 10 minutes.

6. Transfer the chicken to a serving platter. Raise the heat to high and boil the sauce, uncovered, until it has thickened, about 10 minutes. Stir in the cilantro or mint. Spoon the sauce over the chicken to serve.

NOTE: If you have a large preserved lemon (or 2 small ones) on hand, feel free to skip the blanching step and use that instead.

Oven-Roasted Pork Butt with Rosemary, Garlic, and Black Pepper

1 (5- to 7-pound) boneless pork shoulder
4 fat garlic cloves, minced
4 teaspoons kosher salt
1/4 cup extra-virgin olive oil
2 tablespoons finely chopped fresh rosemary
1 1/2 tablespoons Dijon mustard
1 tablespoon freshly ground black pepper

Time: 15 minutes,
plus at least 2 hours'
marinating and about
3 hours' roasting

Serves 12 to 16

1. Carefully cut away the skin from the pork shoulder, leaving a 1/8-inch layer of fat.
2. Using a mortar and pestle or the flat side of a knife, mash together the garlic and salt to form a paste. Stir in the olive oil, rosemary, mustard, and black pepper. Rub the mixture all over the pork and transfer to a large roasting pan. Cover tightly with plastic wrap and refrigerate for at least 2 hours or overnight.
3. Preheat the oven to 325°F and let the pork come to room temperature. Place the pork on a roasting rack fitted inside a roasting pan, skin side up. Roast, uncovered, until the meat is fork-tender (and reaches 180°F on a meat thermometer), 3 to 4 hours. Let rest at least 10 minutes before slicing and serving.

Caramelized Onion and Radicchio Quiche

1 recipe Perfect Piecrust (see page 386)

Time: 1 hour and
25 minutes

Serves 8

1 large egg white
3 tablespoons grated Gruyère cheese (about 3/4 ounce)
3 tablespoons extra-virgin olive oil
1 large red onion, halved and thinly sliced

1¼ teaspoons kosher salt

¼ teaspoon sugar

1 medium radicchio, halved and thinly sliced (about 8 ounces)

1 teaspoon balsamic vinegar

3 large eggs

1½ cups heavy cream

¼ teaspoon freshly grated nutmeg

½ teaspoon freshly ground black pepper

1 tablespoon unsalted butter, cubed

Pinch fleur de sel

1. Preheat the oven to 375°F. On a lightly floured surface, roll the dough to a ³/₈-inch thickness and press into a 9-inch pie pan. Line the dough with foil and fill with pie weights, rice, or dried beans. Bake for 20 minutes, then remove the weights and foil and bake for an additional 5 to 7 minutes, until lightly golden.

2. Take the crust out of the oven and brush the bottom of the crust with the egg white and sprinkle on the Gruyère in an even layer. Return the crust to the oven and bake for 10 to 13 minutes, until lightly browned.

3. Meanwhile, in a large pan, heat 2 tablespoons of oil over medium heat. Add the onion, ½ teaspoon salt, and sugar and cook, stirring occasionally, until the onion is soft and browned, about 15 minutes.

4. Stir in the radicchio and the remaining tablespoon oil and ¼ teaspoon salt and cook, stirring constantly, until the radicchio is very wilted and jammy, about 10 minutes. Stir in the balsamic vinegar and cook 1 minute more.

5. In a medium bowl, whisk together the eggs, cream, nutmeg, the remaining ³/₄ teaspoon salt, and pepper.

6. When the crust is lightly browned and the cheese is melted, sprinkle on ½ cup of the radicchio-onion mixture and carefully pour in the custard. Dot the top with the butter pieces, sprinkle on the fleur de sel, and return to the oven. Bake for 25 to 35 minutes, until the top of the quiche is puffed up and golden and the middle is almost set. Allow the quiche to cool slightly, about 10 minutes, before serving with the remaining radicchio-onion mixture sprinkled on top.

One-Handed Macaroni
with Creamy Peas and Cheese

Kosher salt

8 ounces macaroni or tiny shells pasta (2 cups)

2/3 cup frozen peas

2/3 cup heavy cream

2 large sage sprigs

1 fat garlic clove, minced

1/2 teaspoon freshly grated lemon zest (optional)

1/2 cup grated Parmesan cheese, more to taste

1/4 teaspoon freshly grated nutmeg

Pinch freshly ground black pepper

Time: 10 minutes

Serves 2 adults
or numerous
small children

1. In a large pot of salted water, cook the pasta according to the package directions. About 30 seconds before the pasta is done to taste, stir in the frozen peas. Drain well.
2. While the pasta is cooking, in a medium saucepan, bring the cream, sage, garlic, and lemon zest (if using) to a simmer for about 3 minutes. Stir in the cheese, nutmeg, pepper, pasta, and peas. Stir well until the pasta is coated with the sauce and season with salt to taste. Serve hot, discarding the sage.

My Mother's Crispy Potato Kugel
with Rosemary and Fried Shallots

6 large russet potatoes, peeled and quartered

2 yellow onions, peeled and quartered

5 large eggs

1/4 cup all-purpose flour

1/2 cup extra-virgin olive oil

Time: 1 1/2 hours

Serves 6

2½ teaspoons kosher salt, plus additional for seasoning

2 teaspoons freshly ground black pepper

2 teaspoons finely chopped fresh rosemary

2 garlic cloves, finely chopped

3 shallots, peeled and thinly sliced crosswise

1. Preheat the oven to 400°F.
2. Fit a food processor with a medium grating blade. With the motor running, alternate pushing the potato and onion chunks through the feed tube. Transfer the mixture to a dish towel–lined colander. Wrap the mixture in the towel and squeeze out as much excess liquid as possible.
3. In a large bowl, whisk together the eggs, flour, ¼ cup oil, salt, pepper, rosemary, and garlic.
4. Heat 1 tablespoon of the remaining oil in a 9-inch, slope-sided skillet. Add the shallots in a single layer over high heat. Let sit several minutes before stirring. Continue to cook, stirring occasionally, until the shallots are crispy and dark brown, about 7 minutes total.
5. Fold the potato mixture and shallots in the egg mixture. Return the skillet to high heat and add the remaining 3 tablespoons oil. Tilt the skillet to grease the bottom and sides of the pan. Carefully press the potato mixture into the pan. Cook over high heat for 3 minutes (this will help sear the bottom crust of the kugel). Transfer the pan to the oven and bake until the potatoes are tender and the top of the kugel is golden brown, 1 to 1¼ hours.
6. Place the kugel under the broiler for 1 to 2 minutes to form a crisp crust on top (watch carefully to see that it does not burn). Run an offset spatula around the edges and bottom of the kugel and carefully invert it onto a large plate or platter. Sprinkle with salt and serve.

My Mother's Lemon Pot Roast

6 garlic cloves

1½ tablespoons plus a pinch kosher salt, more to taste

1 (4½-pound) beef brisket

1 teaspoon freshly ground black pepper

3 lemons

½ cup extra-virgin olive oil

Time: 30 minutes,
plus 3 hours' cooking

Serves 10 to 12

1. Mince 1 garlic clove. Using a mortar and pestle or the flat side of a heavy knife, pound or mash the garlic with a pinch of salt until it turns to a paste.

2. Season the brisket all over with salt and pepper and rub the garlic paste into the meat. Place the brisket in a large bowl or pan, cover tightly with plastic wrap, and refrigerate for at least 2 hours or overnight.

3. When you are ready to cook the brisket, preheat the oven to 325°F.

4. Finely grate the zest of 2 lemons and reserve; juice all 3 lemons.

5. Heat the oil in a 6½-quart Dutch oven until almost smoking. Sear the brisket in the oil until browned on all sides, about 10 minutes. Pour the lemon juice over the brisket and add enough water to come halfway up the sides of the meat (about 2 cups). Bring the liquid to a boil over high heat.

6. Cover the pot, transfer to the oven, and cook for 1¼ hours. Meanwhile, mince the remaining 5 garlic cloves. Turn the meat over in the pot and add the garlic. Continue to cook until the meat shreds easily with a fork, about 1 to 1¼ hours longer. Stir in the reserved lemon zest and continue to cook, uncovered, 15 minutes more.

7. Slice and serve, with the pan juices spooned over the meat. Or let cool and refrigerate for up to 5 days before reheating and serving.

Sesame Halvah Toffee

Time: 30 minutes

Makes about
24 pieces

1½ cups all-purpose flour

½ teaspoon kosher salt

10 tablespoons unsalted butter, cubed

2 tablespoons tahini

2 tablespoons sesame seeds, plus additional for sprinkling

1 tablespoon vanilla extract

Demerara (raw) sugar, for sprinkling (optional)

4 ounces dark chocolate, chopped (optional)

3 ounces halvah, crumbled (optional)

1. Preheat the oven to 325°F. In the bowl of a food processor, pulse together the flour and salt just to combine. Add the butter, tahini, sesame seeds, and vanilla. Pulse together until a crumbly dough forms.

2. Press the dough into an 8×8-inch baking dish and smooth the top with a spatula. Use a fork to pierce the top of the dough. (If not using the chocolate, sprinkle the dough generously with the Demerara sugar and additional sesame seeds.) Bake until the top is light golden brown, 20 to 25 minutes.

3. If not using the chocolate, transfer the pan to a wire rack to cool. Otherwise, scatter the chocolate pieces on top of the shortbread. Turn off the heat and return the pan to the oven for 1 to 2 minutes to soften the chocolate. Using an offset spatula, spread the softened chocolate into an even layer over the shortbread. Sprinkle with the crumbled halvah, if using, and allow to cool to room temperature in the pan before cutting.

Salted Maple Walnut Thumbprints

3 cups all-purpose flour
1 teaspoon kosher salt
1 cup (2 sticks) unsalted butter, room temperature
1 cup sugar
1 cup pure maple syrup
2 large egg yolks
12 ounces walnut halves
Fleur de sel or other coarse sea salt, for sprinkling (or use freshly
    grated nutmeg)

Time: 25 minutes,
plus cooling time

Makes 42 cookies

1. Preheat the oven to 350°F. In a medium bowl, whisk together the flour and kosher salt. In the bowl of an electric mixer fitted with the paddle attachment, cream together the butter and sugar until light and fluffy. Scrape down the sides of the bowl, add ½ cup of maple syrup and the egg yolks, and beat until fully incorporated. Add the flour mixture and mix until just combined.

2. Using a tablespoon, drop the dough, 3 inches apart, onto two baking sheets. Using your thumb, make an indentation in the center of each round of dough. Bake until the edges are just golden, 12 to 15 minutes. Transfer to a wire rack to cool.

3. While the cookies are cooling, prepare the maple glaze. Place the remaining ½ cup maple syrup in a small saucepan over medium heat. Simmer the syrup until reduced to about ⅓ cup, 7 to 10 minutes. Carefully spoon the glaze into the thumbprint of each cooled cookie, then place a walnut and a sprinkle of salt (or nutmeg) on top. Allow the glaze to set, at least 10 minutes, before serving.

Kate's Impossibly Fudgy Brownies with Chile and Sea Salt

Time: 45 minutes

Makes 24
(2-inch) squares

2 sticks plus 2 tablespoons unsalted butter

3 ounces unsweetened chocolate, chopped

1 1/2 cups all-purpose flour

1/2 teaspoon kosher salt

1/8 teaspoon cayenne, optional

1/2 cup plus 1 tablespoon cocoa powder

2 1/2 cups sugar

3 large eggs, lightly beaten

1 tablespoon vanilla extract

Maldon salt, for sprinkling

1. Preheat the oven to 350°F. Line a rimmed 9×13-inch baking sheet with parchment paper.
2. In a microwave or in the top bowl of a double boiler, melt together the butter and chopped chocolate, stirring until smooth. Meanwhile, combine the flour, kosher salt, and cayenne in a medium bowl.
3. Transfer the chocolate mixture to a large mixing bowl and whisk in the cocoa powder and sugar. Add the eggs and vanilla; whisk until smooth.
4. Fold in the dry ingredients and continue folding until no lumps remain.
5. Scrape the batter into the prepared pan and smooth the top with a spatula. Sprinkle all over with Maldon salt. Bake for 25 to 30 minutes, until the edges just begin to pull away from the sides of the pan and the top is set and shiny.
6. Allow the brownie to cool completely in the pan before cutting into 2×2-inch squares.

Ridiculously Easy Maple Walnut Ice Cream

2/3 cup maple syrup, preferably Grade B
2 cups heavy cream
2/3 cup whole milk
Large pinch kosher salt
3/4 cup chopped toasted walnuts

Time: 10 minutes
plus freezing time

Makes 1 1/2 pints

1. In a large saucepan over medium heat, bring the maple syrup just to a boil. Reduce the heat to low and simmer to thicken for 5 minutes.
2. Take the pan off the heat and whisk in the cream, milk, and salt. Transfer the mixture to a bowl to cool to room temperature, then chill until quite cold, at least 1 hour and up to 2 days.
3. Freeze the mixture in an ice-cream maker according to the manufacturer's directions. When the ice cream is almost at the desired consistency, stir in the nuts and continue freezing another 5 minutes. Transfer the ice cream to an airtight container and store in the freezer.

Twenty-Ingredient Pie (Spiced Apple-Pear-Cranberry Crumb Pie)

1 recipe Perfect Piecrust (see recipe, page 386)
1/2 cup golden raisins
1/2 cup dark raisins
1/3 cup dark rum
2/3 cup dark brown sugar
2 apples (about 1 pound), peeled, cored, and cut into 1/2-inch slices
2 large pears (about 1 pound), peeled, cored, and cut into 1/2-inch slices
2/3 cup fresh or frozen cranberries
3 tablespoons granulated sugar
2 tablespoons cornstarch
2 tablespoons freshly squeezed lemon juice

Time: 90 minutes

Serves 6 to 8

½ teaspoon ground cinnamon

¼ teaspoon ground ginger

¼ teaspoon freshly grated nutmeg

Pinch kosher salt

FOR THE CRUMB TOPPING

½ cup all-purpose flour

½ cup rolled oats

½ cup light brown sugar

¼ cup chopped toasted walnuts

1 teaspoon ground cinnamon

½ teaspoon freshly grated nutmeg

¼ teaspoon kosher salt

½ cup (1 stick) unsalted butter, chilled and cubed

1. On a lightly floured surface or between two sheets of plastic wrap, roll the pie dough into a ³/₈-inch-thick round. Line a 9-inch pie pan with the dough, use your thumb and forefinger to flute the edges, and chill in the refrigerator while you prepare the filling (or for up to 1 day; lightly cover the dough with plastic if leaving for more than 2 hours).

2. In a medium saucepan over medium-high heat, combine the raisins and rum with ⅓ cup water. Stir in the brown sugar and bring to a boil. Simmer, stirring occasionally, until the sugar is dissolved, then remove from the heat, cover, and let cool to room temperature.

3. In a large bowl, combine the apples, pears, cranberries, granulated sugar, cornstarch, lemon juice, cinnamon, ginger, nutmeg, and salt. When the raisin mixture has cooled, scrape it into the fruit mixture, tossing well to combine. Allow the fruit mixture to rest at room temperature while you bake the crust.

4. Preheat the oven to 375°F. Line the crust with foil, fill with pie weights, and place on a foil-lined baking sheet. Bake the crust until light golden brown, about 20 minutes. Take the pan out of the oven and remove the foil and weights.

[CONTINUED]

5. Scrape the filling into the crust, piling the fruit into a mound in the center so it does not spill out. Return the pie to the oven and bake for 30 minutes.

6. Meanwhile, prepare the crumb topping. In a medium bowl, mix together the flour, oats, brown sugar, nuts, cinnamon, nutmeg, and salt. Using your fingers, rub the butter into the flour mixture until large crumbs form. Carefully remove the pie from the oven and sprinkle the crumb topping all over the filling. Return the pie to the oven and bake until the fruit is very tender and the juices are bubbling, another 30 to 35 minutes. Check after 20 minutes; if the crumb topping looks too brown, tent the pie with a sheet of foil. Allow the pie to cool for 25 to 30 minutes on a wire rack before serving.

Perfect Piecrust

1 1/4 cups all-purpose flour
1/4 teaspoon kosher salt
10 tablespoons unsalted butter, preferably a high-fat, European-style butter such as Plugra, chilled, and cut into 1/2-inch pieces
2 to 5 tablespoons ice water

1. In a food processor, briefly pulse together the flour and salt. Add the butter and pulse until the mixture forms chickpea-size pieces (3 to 5 1-second pulses). Add the ice water, 1 tablespoon at a time, and pulse until the mixture is just moist enough to hold together.

2. Form the dough into a ball, wrap with plastic, and flatten into a disc. Refrigerate at least 1 hour before rolling out and baking.

Time: 15 minutes, plus chilling time

Makes 1 (9-inch) single piecrust; recipe can be doubled for a double crust; divide the dough into two balls to form two discs before chilling.

Index